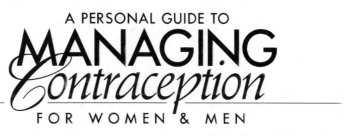

A PERSONAL GUIDE TO
MANAGING
Contraception
FOR WOMEN & MEN

Edition for the year 2000

Robert A. Hatcher, MD, MPH
Professor of Gynecology and Obstetrics
Emory University School of Medicine

Erika I. Pluhar
PhD Candidate, Human Sexuality Education
University of Pennsylvania

Miriam Zieman, MD
Assistant Professor of Gynecology and Obstetrics
Emory University School of Medicine

Anita L. Nelson, MD
Professor of Obstetrics and Gynecology
University of California Los Angeles School of Medicine

Philip D. Darney, MD, MSc
Professor of Obstetrics, Gynecology and Reproductive Sciences
San Francisco General Hospital
University of California, San Francisco

Alston Parker Watt, MPH
Research Assistant
Department of Gynecology and Obstetrics
Emory University School of Medicine

Peter W. Hatcher, MD
Family Physician
Multnomah County Health Department, Portland, Oregon

Technical and Computer Support:
Anna Poyner, Don Bagwell, Max Harrell, Bill Stratton
and Digital Impact Design, Inc, Cornelia, Georgia

FYI: *As of February 29, 2000, we have provided 164,000 free copies of the companion pocket guide, **Managing Contraception**, to medical students, physicians (particularly residents), nurses, nursing students, nurse practitioners, and physician assistants. Most of these copies were provided through a grant from the David and Lucile Packard Foundation. Copies were also given away by Organon, Parke Davis, and Wyeth Pharmaceutical companies. Total sales and distribution by June 2000 (when the new edition of the **Pocket Guide** comes out) will be 250,000 books.*

Bridging the Gap Communications, Inc.   Dawsonville, Georgia & Tiger, Georgia

COPYRIGHT INFORMATION

DISCLAIMER

The authors advise the reader to consult a primary-care clinician or a specialist
in obstetrics, gynecology, or urology (depending on the contraceptive method
or condition); the package insert; or other references, before making decisions
about managing or treating any problem. Under no circumstances should the
reader use this book instead of—or to override—the judgment of the treating
clinician. The authors and staff are not liable for errors or omissions.

Edition for the year 2000
ISBN 0-9671939-2-3
Printed in the United States of America
Bridging the Gap, Communication Inc.
www.managingcontraception.com

TABLE OF CONTENTS

*Devoted to the
reproductive health
and happiness of
women and men...*

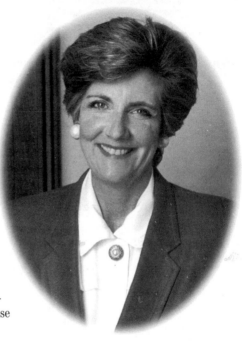

Sharon Camp's professional life has been devoted to the reproductive health and happiness of women and men. On *60 Minutes*, *The Today Show* and *Good Morning America* as well as 60 other national television appearances she has advocated for women's rights to choose and explained and fought for contraceptive options. Her efforts have borne fruit in the United States, Europe and throughout the world.

Sharon L. Camp Ph.D.

Dr. Camp has been Chair of the Board of Family Health International, the International Center for Research on Women, and the National Council for International Health. For 18 years she was Senior Vice President of Population Action International.

Sharon was an honors graduate of Pomona College in California. She holds Masters and Doctoral degrees in comparative and international politics from Johns Hopkins University.

Her most recent and perhaps most ambitious effort has been to bring to couples in the United States the emergency contraceptive pill called *Plan B*. For this and all the many blessings your life has brought to the reproductive health community and to women and families, we thank you heartily, Sharon.

So many have contributed their sensitivity, time, graphics and layout skills, financial support, friendship, encouragement, patience and love in the creation of *Managing Contraception* and this companion book for the general public, *A Personal Guide to Managing Contraception.* All of our parents helped us strive to be the very best that we can be and aided us along the way. These two books contain the best that we have to offer— the very best way we know to communicate, one in a format that clinicians and counselors can carry and refer to easily, and the other in a format that women and men considering contraceptive options can use. Gems have come to us from many corners. We thank all contributors, including:

- **Jeffrey Allen,** radiologist in Atlanta and artist in residence
- **Felix Andarsio,** a fine resident in obstetrics and gynecology at Emory University
- **Marcia Ann Angle,** committed international leader in the quest for high quality reproductive health services at INTRAH at the University of North Carolina (UNC), Chapel Hill
- **Anne Atkinson,** training advisor at JHPIEGO; nurse midwifery student at Georgetown; one of tomorrow's leaders
- **Leslie Banta**, law librarian for Womble Carlyle in Atlanta, GA
- **Jim Bellinger,** PA at Grady Memorial Hospital in Atlanta; extraordinary attention to detail
- **Audra Bernstein,** first-year curriculum coordinator, Cornell University Medical College
- **Rachel Blankstein,** author of pilot edition of *Managing Contraception* and Peace Corps volunteer in Niger
- **Lynn Borgatta,** medical abortion researcher; OB/GYN faculty at Boston University; wife of Gary Stewart, to whom *1999 -2000 Pocket Guide to Managing Contraception* is dedicated
- **Paige Bossi**, physician assistant in obstetrics and gynecology at Grady Memorial Hospital
- **Stephen Brandt,** research assistant who coordinated evaluation of *Managing Contraception;* has deep reservoir of concern and caring and great attention to detail; medical student at Wake Forest University
- **Bruce Brown,** public health student at Emory; strong interest in international health
- **Vaughn Bryant,** master's student in marital and family therapy at Northwestern
- **Michael Burnhill,** vice president, Planned Parenthood Federation of America; strong advocate for family planning and reproductive health
- **Martha Campbell** and the David and Lucile Packard Foundation, for making the first two editions of the *Pocket Guide to Managing Contraception* possible
- **Sarah Cates,** medical student at University of North Carolina, Chapel Hill. Watch her, world, here comes a great one!
- **Willard Cates,** president, Family Health International, researcher in contraception, STIs, and HIV, and an author of *Contraceptive Technology*; cheerleader!
- **Camaryn Chrisman,** pre-med student; very helpful in evaluation of *Managing Contraception*
- **Julie Clark,** Cornell medical student, with a sensitive approach to the contraceptives we write about in this book
- **Claudette Colestock,** child and family therapist in Westchester, PA
- **Shannon Colestock,** health and sexuality educator Westtown School, Westtown, PA
- **Raul A. Cortes,** graduating Emory medical student with incredible suggestions
- **Mitchell D. Creinin,** researcher on emergency contraception, medical abortion, Magee-Womens Hospital (University of Pittsburgh Health Center)
- **Sally Faith Dorfman,** director of the Division of Public Health and Education for the Medical Society of New York
- **Susan Eisendrath,** reproductive health director at the American Medical Women's Association
- **Kim Bailey Fortner,** graduate of the University of Tennessee, third-year Emory medical student and future OB/GYN
- **Erica Frank,** writer, editor and assistant professor of family and preventive medicine at Emory
- **Yvonne Fulbright,** sexuality educator and Director of the National AIDS Fund Fellowship Program, American Medical Student Association

- **Meera Garcia,** Emory resident in OB/GYN; one of this world's truly enthusiastic people!
- **Eric Garrison,** health educator at the University of Baltimore, MD
- **Felicia Guest,** AIDS educator, wise observer, and an author of *Contraceptive Technology*
- **John Guillebaud,** professor of family planning and reproductive health at University College London Hospitals and medical director of the Margaret Pyke Center for Study and Training in Family Planning. We thank John for permission to use information from *Contraception Today* (Martin Dunitz Ltd., London) in *Managing Contraception*
- **Kristen Harvey,** student at Cornell University Medical College; wonderful editor
- **Arminda Hicks,** state family planning coordinator for Georgia
- **Van Hoo,** Emory University graduate leaning toward the Peace Corps and a career in public health
- **Margie Hutchison,** sensitive artist in Atlanta
- **Andrew Kaunitz,** professor and assistant chair, department of OB/GYN, University of Florida Health Sciences Center, Jacksonville, Florida
- **Maxine Keel,** administrative assistant at the Emory University Family Planning Program, dreamer, inspiration and friend
- **Maggie Kelly,** student, humorist at the University of Georgia in Athens
- **Holly Kennedy,** Director, Graduate Program in Nurse-Midwifery at the University of Rhode Island; a thoughtful and thorough review of *A Personal Guide* has greatly improved the book
- **Victor LaCerva,** inspiring speaker, Family Health Bureau Medical Director, New Mexico Department of Health
- **Anne Mather,** editor, writer and wise mother of Maggie Kelly
- **Monica McGrann**, medical student with indomitable enthusiasm, Texas A&M
- **Radhika Mohan,** University of Washington student, wrote & edited chapters in *Managing Contraception* and is pictured teaching the pill danger signals (on right, page 125)
- **Veronica E. Murillo,** director of health education; Education Programs Associates, Campbell, CA
- **Bert Peterson,** contraceptive research leader at Centers for Disease Control in Atlanta and at the World Health Organization in Geneva; professor of gynecology at Emory
- **Anna Poyner,** graphic artist who designed this book; Digital Impact Design, Inc. in Cornelia, Georgia
- **Kanishka Ratanayaka,** Emory medical student
- **Mary Rosser,** former resident in OB/GYN at Emory University; OB/GYN in Westchester, NY
- **Sharon Schnare,** consultant and trainer in Seattle; remarkable teacher, dreamer
- **Kristin Schofield,** resident in family medicine at UNC-Chapel Hill
- **Tara Shochet,** PhD candidate at the Office of Population Research at Princeton University
- **Ari Silverstein,** meticulous and creative Emory medical student
- **Renda Soylemez,** Columbia University medical student, going into OB/GYN
- **Hallie Stosur,** creative and caring physician trained in OB/GYN, Oregon Health Sciences University in Portland, Oregon; clinician at Kaiser Permanente in Portland
- **Christian Thrasher,** Health Education Program Director for 100 Black Men of America in Atlanta, GA
- **Andrea Tone,** historian in the Department of History, Technology and Society at Georgia Tech, Atlanta; specializes in the history of contraception
- **James Trussell,** an author of *Contraceptive Technology* who developed the failure rates and cost figures used throughout *Managing Contraception;* remarkable attention to detail
- **Marcel Vekemans,** family planning specialist from Belgium; now at INTRAH
- **Jane Wamsher,** nurse practitioner at Grady Memorial Hospital in Atlanta; provided practical protocols and creative techniques for using book to teach
- **Lee Warner,** CDC researcher working on STIs and HIV; excellent help on the condom chapters
- **Elisa S. Wells,** senior program officer at PATH; emergency contraception expert
- **Ssu Weng,** Title X medical director for New Mexico; excellent editor
- **Anna Willingham,** women's health advocate; Executive Director, Georgia STD Prevention Coalition; photographed demonstrating the pill danger signals (on left, page 125)
- **Sue Willis,** nurse living in Clayton, GA
- **Janet Witte,** Middlebury College graduate and student in Emory University's MD/MPH program
- **Anne Zweifel,** fine resident in OB/GYN at UNC-Chapel Hill

You have in your hands a compilation of important contraceptive and family planning information. This book is derived directly from another hand book for physicians, nurses, physician's assistants, nurse practitioners, and nurse-midwives. For people trying to use contraception safely and effectively, we hope you find this book helpful.

The book is organized in large part around the concept of the advantages and disadvantages of each approach to birth control. No contraceptive is perfect. It may be expensive, difficult to use, or have a relatively high rate of failure. It may have important side effects or potential complications. All these negatives are outlined on the pages of this book.

The advantages of each method are also presented. More and more emphasis is being placed on the noncontraceptive benefits of each contraceptive. Birth control pills prevent ovarian cancer, endometrial cancer and benign (non-cancerous) breast lumps. Pills decrease painful periods (the number one cause of missed work in women ages 20-50). In addition, pills may be used to treat acne. Depo-Provera is widely used in the treatment of endometriosis. Tubal sterilization decreases a woman's risk for pelvic infection and ovarian cancer.

Half of all pregnancies in the United States are unplanned or unintended. Many are unwanted. For every 1000 infants born there are 340 abortions. These are sobering statistics for our seemingly advanced nation. We can interact instantly around the globe with cellular phones and wireless internet devices, but we have such a tough time having sexual intercourse without often tragic outcomes. Why? What's behind the failure? There are probably many answers. The two most important answers, we feel, are: (1) that contraception is a low priority in terms of education, public dialogue, research, and service in our society and (2) that sexual intimacy is difficult for individuals and for our society to deal with rationally, carefully, deliberately and responsibly.

Perhaps this little book will help men and women, sexually active adolescents, and all hoping to avoid unintended pregnancy and infection to use prevention methods as close to perfectly as possible. Please share this book with your family and friends!

The future of contraception is exciting. Birth control will change so much. Save this book for your children and grandchildren, who might like to be able to look back on how things were in the year 2000!

Photo Day for Managing Contraception

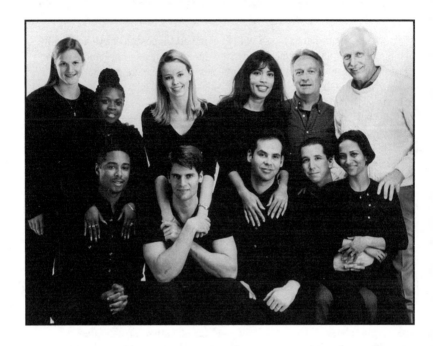

From the left, top row: Erika Pluhar, author and Ph.D. Candidate in Human Sexuality Education at the University of Pennsylvania; LaChelle Keel; Donelle Martin; Odalys Andarsio; John Stanley, publisher and distributor, Bridging the Gap Communications, Inc.; and Bob Hatcher, Professor of gynecology and obstetrics at Emory University and President of the Bridging the Gap Foundation. From the left, bottom row: Eric Keel; Henry Millwood; Felix Andarsio; Paul Garcia; and Meera Garcia.

Each of the couples to the right is pictured throughout the book accompanied by a story, real-life example, or message related to family planning and contraception. The photos are placed immediately before the chapter to which they are related. For example, go to the pages before the Sexually Transmitted Infection chapter to learn 99 ways to be sexual and stay infection-free.

Meet the Couples Pictured In This Book

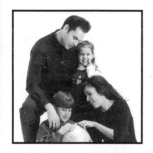

FELIX AND ODALYS ANDARSIO
Felix and Odalys are married and have two beautiful children, Zoey and Emmanuel. Felix is the chief resident in gynecology and obstetrics at Emory University. Before becoming a full-time mom, Odalys worked in the field of real estate management.

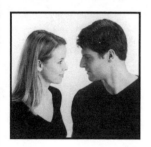

DONELLE MARTIN AND HENRY MILLWOOD
Donelle and Henry have been together for over a year. Donelle graduated from nursing school at the Medical College of Georgia. Henry is a medical student at the Medical College of Georgia.

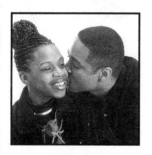

ERIC AND LACHELLE KEEL
Eric and Lachelle Keel are married and the proud parents of one-year-old Marquis. Eric is an employee of the Mead Corporation and Lachelle is a student at Georgia Medical Institution and a part-time employee at Service Master Aviation. They plan to get pregnant again when Marquis is five.

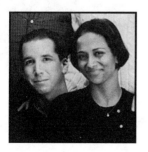

MEERA AND PAUL GARCIA
Meera and Paul are married and are the proud new parents of Violet. Meera is a resident in gynecology and obstetrics at Emory University and Paul is an M.D./Ph.D. student, also at Emory. His Ph.D. will be in bioengineering from a joint program with Georgia Tech.

1. Keep it in a handy place. Share it with others!

2. The contraceptive method chapters present complete, up-to-date information on the advantages and disadvantages of each method. Use these chapters to learn about methods, help you choose a method, identify possible side effects and benefits, and to teach others.

3. Women and men who are having sex MUST be concerned about sexually transmitted infections. We have included pages 158-179 to give you the information you need to prevent, recognize, and get treated for infections.

4. Color photos of pills will help you to determine the pills you may have used and are using (pages 117-124).

5. The pages on the menstrual cycle explain a very complicated process. We have tried to make it as simple as possible to help readers understand this important part of female physiology.

6. Flowcharts that might help you are:
   • Page   52: How to use a latex condom
   • Page 104: How to choose a pill
   • Page 109: What to do about breakthrough bleeding or spotting on pills
   • Page 111: What to do if you miss a pill
   • Page 132: What to do if you are late for your Depo-Provera shot
   • Page 152: What to do if you are in your early 20s and want tubal sterilization

AIDS	Acquired immunodeficiency syndrome	**IPPF**	International Planned Parenthood Federation
ASAP	As soon as possible	**IUD**	Intrauterine device
AZT	Azidothymidine, ZDV	**IV**	Intravenous
BBT	Basal body temperature	**LAM**	Lactation amenorrhea method
BSE	Breast self-examination	**LDL**	Low-density lipoprotein
BTB	Breakthrough bleeding (vaginal)	**LH**	Luteinizing hormone
BV	Bacterial vaginosis	**MTX**	Methotrexate
CDC	Centers for Disease Control and Prevention	**N/A**	Not applicable
		NFP	Natural family planning
COCs	Combined oral contraceptives	**NGU**	Nongonococcal urethritis
D & C	Dilation and curettage	**N-9**	Nonoxynol-9
DMPA	Depo-Provera	**O-9**	Octoxynol-9
EC	Emergency contraception	**OB/GYN**	Obstetrics & Gynecology
ECPs	Emergency contraceptive pills ("morning-after pills")	**OC**	Oral contraceptive
		Pap	Papanicolaou (pap test)
EMS	Emergency medical services	**PID**	Pelvic inflammatory disease
ER	Emergency Room	**PMS**	Premenstrual syndrome
ERT	Estrogen replacement therapy, includes estrogen and progesterone treatments	**POPs**	Progestin-only pill (minipill)
		PPFA	Planned Parenthood Federation of America
FAM	Fertility awareness methods	**RTI**	Reproductive tract infection
FDA	Food and Drug Administration	**STI**	Sexually transmissible infection
FSH	Follicle stimulating hormone		
GnRH	Gonadotropin-releasing hormone	**TB**	Tuberculosis
		TL	Tubal ligation
HCG	Human chorionic gonadotrophin	**TSS**	Toxic shock syndrome
		UTI	Urinary tract infection
HDL	High density lipoprotein	**VCF**	Vaginal Contraceptive Film
HIV	Human immunodeficiency virus	**VSC**	Voluntary surgical contraception
HPV	Human papilloma virus	**WHO**	World Health Organization
HRT	Hormone replacement therapy		
HSV	Herpes simplex virus		

TOPIC	ORGANIZATION	WEBSITE
Abortion	National Abortion Rights Action League	www.naral.org
	National Abortion Federation	www.prochoice.org/naf
Adolescent Reproductive Health	National Campaign to Prevent Teen Pregnancy	www.teenpregnancy.org
	Advocates for Youth	www.advocatesforyouth.org
	Coalition for Positive Sexuality	www.positive.org
	American Medical Association	www.ama-assn.org/adolhlth
Adoption	National Adoption Center	www.nac.adopt.org
	National Adoption Information Clearinghouse	www.calib.org/naic
Breastfeeding	La Leche League	www.lalecheleague.org
	Breastfeeding.com	www.breastfeeding.com
Contraception	Bridging the Gap Communications, Inc. (publishes this book)	www.managingcontraception.com
	Planned Parenthood Federation of America	www.plannedparenthood.org
	International Planned Parenthood Federation	www.ippf.org
	Contraceptive and Research Development Program	www.conrad.org
	Johns Hopkins University affiliate corporation	www.jhpiego.jhu.edu
	Centers for Disease Control	www.cdc.gov
	Association for Voluntary Surgical Contraception	www.avsc.org
Emergency Contraception	Office of Population Research/Princeton University	www.opr.princeton.edu
Gay/Lesbian/Bisexual/Transgender	Gay Men's Health Crisis	www.gmhc.org
	Human Rights Campaign	www.hrc.org
	Youth Assistance Organization	www.youth.org
	Parents and Friends of Gays and Lesbians	www.pflag.org
	National Gay and Lesbian Task Force	www.ngltf.org
	Pridenet	www.pridenet.com
Healthcare Professionals	American Academy of Family Physicians	www.aafp.org
	American College of Nurse-Midwives	www.acnm.org
	American College of Obstetrics and Gynecology	www.acog.org

TOPIC	ORGANIZATION	WEBSITE
Healthcare Professionals (cont.)	Association of Reproductive Health Professionals	www.ahrp.org
	Federal Drug Administration	www.fda.gov
	Planned Parenthood Federation of America	www.plannedparenthood.org
	American Medical Association	www.ama-assn.org
HIV/AIDS/	Centers for Disease Control	www.cdc.gov/nchstp
Sexually Transmitted Infections	American Social Health Association	www.ashastd.org
	American Herpes Foundation	www.herpes-foundation.org
	Critical Path AIDS Project	www.critpath.org
	American Foundation for AIDS Research	www.amfar.org
	National Association of People with AIDS	www.thecure.org
Menopause	North American Menopause Society	www.menopause.org
Natural Family Planning	California Family Health Council	www.cfhc.org
	University of Southern California	www.usc.edu/hsc/info/newman/resource/nfp.html
Population	Population Council	www.popcouncil.org
	Population Reference Bureau	www.prb.org
	United Nations Development Programme	www.undp.org
	Population Communications International	www.population.org
Reproductive Health Research	Alan Guttmacher Institute	www.agi-usa.org
	Kaiser Family Foundation	www.kff.org
	Family Health International	www.fhi.org
Sexual Assault/Domestic Violence	Sexual Assault Information Page	www.cs.utk.edu/~bartley/saInfoPage.html
	U.S. Department of Justice	www.ojp.usdoj.gov/vawo/
	Family Violence Awareness Page	www.famvi.com
Sexual Health/Sexualtiy Education	Sexuality Information and Education Council for the U.S.	www.siecus.org
	Sexual Health Network	www.sexualhealth.com
	Safer Sex Institute	www.safersex.org

TOPIC	ORGANIZATION	PHONE NUMBER
Abortion	Abortion Hotline (National Abortion Federation)	800-772-9100
Abuse/Rape	National Committee to Prevent Child Abuse	312-663-3520
	National Resource Center on Violence	800-537-2238
	Centers for Disease Control Rape Hotline	800-656-4673
	Spanish	800-344-7432
		800-243-7889
Adoption	Adopt a Special Kid-America	202-388-3888
	Adoptive Families of America	612-535-4829
Breastfeeding	La Leche League	800-LA-LECHE
Contraception	Planned Parenthood	800-230-7526
	Family Health International	919-544-7040
	Planned Parenthood Federation of America	212-541-7800
Counseling	Peer Counseling for Gay/Lesbian/Bisexual	800-969-6884
	Peer Listening Line Gay/Lesbian/Bisexual	800-399-7337
	Depression after Delivery	800-944-4773
Emergency Contraception	Emergency Contraception Information	888-NOT-2-LATE
		888-PREVEN2
HIV/AIDS	Centers for Disease Control AIDS Hotline	800-342-2437
	Centers for Disease Control	
	National AIDS Clearinghouse	800-458-5231
	AIDS Clinical Trials Information Service	800-874-2572
	Gay Men's Health Crisis	800-AIDS-NYC
Pregnancy	National Pregnancy Hotline	800-311-2229
	Lamaze International	800-368-4404
STIs	Hepatitis B Coalition	612-647-9009
	Centers for Disease Control	
	Sexually Transmitted Disease Hotline	800-227-8922
	Herpes and HPV Hotline	800-230-6039

Before we proceed to the formal chapters in this book, a note of caution about having intercourse without having it lead to an unintended pregnancy. Small mistakes can prove costly. Failure to withdraw in time; using condoms 99 out of 100 times; missing pills; starting packages of pills 3 days too late; failure to detect a partially expelled IUD; or having unprotected sex the night before a tubal sterilization all may lead to an unintended pregnancy which may change the entire course of a person or couple's life.

The woman who takes her pill the very first thing each morning AND notes this with a red check in her daily calendar AND has the man in her life call daily to check—did you take the pill and jot it down on the calendar?—is on her way to extremely effective oral contraceptive use. She may also have a rule for herself that she always has at least one full cycle of pills in her medicine chest and usually buys 6 cycles of pills at a time. She thinks of her pills as a form of therapy—preventative medicine against the risk of an unintended pregnancy.

We encourage readers to be compulsive in this area of life. The prevention of unintended pregnancy and unwanted infection is what this book is all about. We hope it helps you.

Female Reproductive Anatomy

Know thyself! That is the focus of chapters 1 and 2, where an overview of female and male reproductive anatomy, including detailed diagrams, are provided. Use these sections to answer your own questions, refamiliarize yourself, or teach others.

Side view of internal female reproductive anatomy

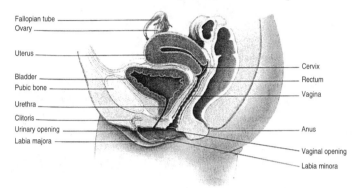

From <u>Human Sexuality: Diversity in Contemporary America, Third Edition</u> by Bryan Strong and Christine DeVault. Copyright 1999 by Mayfield Publishing Company. Reprinted by permission of the publisher.

The internal female reproductive anatomy includes the following:

- ***vagina,*** a muscular structure that serves two reproductive purposes: it encompasses the penis during sexual intercourse and is the passage for a baby during birth. The vagina is lined with mucous membranes that lubricate when a woman is sexually aroused

- ***uterus,*** or womb, is a hollow, muscular organ where a fetus develops during pregnancy. The internal walls of the uterus, or *endometrium,* are rich with tiny blood vessels that fill with blood to prepare for pregnancy (this is where the blood comes from when a woman is not pregnant and has her period)

- ***cervix,*** the opening to the uterus. It has to expand to allow a baby to pass through during birth

- ***urethra,*** the tube through which urine passes from the bladder to the outer part of the vagina

- ***bladder,*** organ that holds urine

- ***ovaries,*** organs on either side of the uterus that produce *ova*, or eggs, the female reproductive cells. Also produce the female hormones estrogen and progesterone; about the size of large almonds

- ***fallopian tubes,*** narrow tubes through which a fertilized egg travels from the ovary to the uterus

Front view of external female genitals

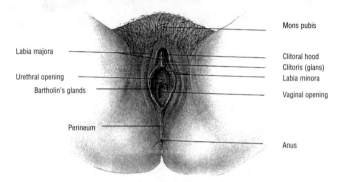

From <u>Human Sexuality: Diversity in Contemporary America, Third Edition</u> by Bryan Strong and Christine DeVault. Copyright 1999 by Mayfield Publishing Company. Reprinted by permission of the publisher.

Together, all of the female external genitals are referred to as the ***vulva***. *The vulva includes the following:*

- ***mons pubis,*** or pubic mound, a pad of fatty tissue that covers the pubic bone and is covered by hair starting at puberty. Sensitive to sexual stimulation in some women

- ***clitoris,*** organ with a high concentration of nerve endings, the only known purpose of which is sexual pleasure. Has external and internal parts—the *glans clitoris*, which is the sensitive tip, is on the outside and is covered by the *clitoral hood*, a fold of skin; and the *clitoral limbre or legs* (not pictured), which extend upward inside the body about 3 inches and contains spongy tissue that fill with blood when a woman is sexually aroused

- ***labia majora,*** or major lips, are two folds of skin that extend from the mons pubis and surround the labia minora, clitoris, urethral opening, and vaginal opening

- ***labia minora,*** or minor lips, two smaller folds of skin that meet to form the clitoral hood and swell during sexual arousal. Every woman's labia minora are different

- ***urethral opening,*** a small hole through which urine flows from the urethra

- ***vaginal opening (or hymen),*** opening leading to the vagina, through which a woman bleeds during her monthly periods and through which a baby passes during birth. In some women, a thin membrane called the hymen covers the vaginal opening. An intact hymen used to be considered evidence of virginity, but it is now known that the hymen can break or stretch before sexual intercourse due to other physical activity or tampon use

Other structures include:

- ***Bartholin's glands***, small glands on either side of the vaginal opening that secrete a small amount of fluid during sexual arousal

- ***anus***, opening to the rectum through which feces is passed. Consists of two sphincters, tight, circular muscles that can be relaxed and contracted. Tissue that surrounds the anus is sexually sensitive in some people

- ***perineum,*** area between the vaginal opening and anus made of soft tissue and sexually sensitive in many people

Male Reproductive Anatomy

Side view of internal male reproductive structures

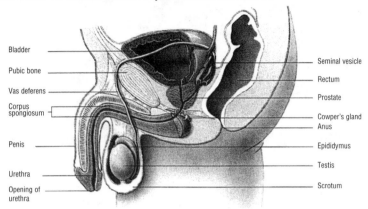

From <u>Human Sexuality: Diversity in Contemporary America, Third Edition</u> by Bryan Strong and Christine DeVault. Copyright 1999 by Mayfield Publishing Company. Reprinted by permission of the publisher.

On the inside, a man has the following reproductive structures:

• **testes,** male reproductive glands. Produce sperm (about 5-10% of ejaculate) and produce and regulate the hormone testosterone

• **epididymus,** stores sperm while they mature

• **vas deferens,** tubes that transport sperm from the epididymus to the seminal vesicle and prostate gland

• **seminal vesicle,** produces a fluid that makes up about 60% of ejaculate

• **prostate gland,** produces about 30-35% of the fluid in ejaculate

• **Cowper's glands,** two small glands below the prostate that connect to the urethra and produce a small amount of fluid before ejaculation (*preejaculatory fluid,* or "precum")

• **bladder,** organ that stores urine

• **urethra,** tube through which urine passes

Other structures include:

• **anus,** the opening from the rectum through which feces passes. Consists of two sphincters tight, circular muscles—that can be relaxed and contracted. Tissue that surrounds the anus is sexually sensitive in some people

Front view of external male genitals

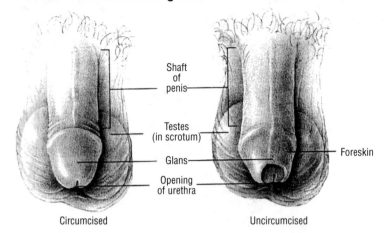

Shaft of penis

Testes (in scrotum)

Glans

Opening of urethra

Foreskin

Circumcised

Uncircumcised

From <u>Human Sexuality: Diversity in Contemporary America, Third Edition</u> by Bryan Strong and Christine DeVault. Copyright 1999 by Mayfield Publishing Company. Reprinted by permission of the publisher.

A man's penis may be circumcised (the foreskin has been removed) or uncircumcised (the foreskin is intact). Depending on whether or not he has been circumcised, the external genitals may look slightly different.

The external genitals contain the following structures:

• **penis,** organ through which sperm pass when a man ejaculates (cums). The penis also contains the urethra, the tube through which urine flows. The penis has three parts: the *root,* the part that attaches to the pelvis, the *shaft,* the body of the penis, and the *glans,* the head of the penis which has the *urethral opening* at its tip. In many men, the underside of the glans is the most sexually sensitive part of the penis because it has a high concentration of nerve endings (similar to the clitoris in a woman). The penis contains the *corpus spongiosum* and *corpus cavernosa,* spongy structures that fill with blood when a man has an erection

• **foreskin,** in an uncircumcised man, a thin layer of skin that covers the penis. It pulls back when the penis becomes erect

• **scrotum,** thin sac-like layer of skin that contains the testicles. The scrotum is attached to a man's body with muscles that contract and relax, pulling the testicles close to the body or releasing them in order to control their temperature

Understanding the Menstrual Cycle

Understanding the menstrual cycle is helpful when discussing contraception because many methods change the physiology of the menstrual cycle to prevent pregnancy. This chapter provides a basic outline of the process to help you better understand your or your partner's body. [Adapted from *Contraceptive Technology*]

- A woman's ovaries make *oocytes* (eggs) as well as the hormones that regulate female reproduction. In contrast to the male reproductive system where large numbers of sperm are produced continuously, a women is born with a set amount of eggs and only one egg is released each month from *menarche* (when a girl starts having periods) to *menopause* (when periods stop)

- During each menstrual cycle, a series of events occurs that ends in *ovulation* (the release of a mature egg) and then the preparation of the *endometrium* (the lining of the uterus) for implantation of a fertilized egg

- The menstrual cycle is regulated by a structure in the brain called the *hypothalamus*, by the nearby pituitary gland, and by the ovaries. These structures send signals and secrete hormones (chemicals carried in the blood stream) that are involved in the monthly development of eggs and the preparation of the uterine lining

- Normal menstrual cycles range from 23 to 35 days, and the cycles of individual women may vary from month to month. Only 15% of women have a consistent 28-day cycle. The three phases of ovarian activity are the *follicular*, *ovulatory*, and *luteal* phases. If a woman does not become pregnant during a cycle, the lining of the uterus is shed and a woman menstruates. As *menstruation* occurs, a new egg begins to develop

PHASES OF THE MENSTRUAL CYCLE

Follicular Phase:
During the first half of the follicular phase, *follicles*, the saclike structures in the ovaries where eggs develop and mature, begin to grow. The hormone *estrogen* sends a signal to another hormone called *follicle-stimulating hormone (FSH)*. FSH "stimulates" the follicles, causing them to grow. At about day 7, a "dominant" follicle emerges and continues to grow while the other follicles stop growing. The dominant follicle continues to produce high levels of estrogen. The length of the follicular phase varies from woman to woman, but it is usually between 10 and 17 days. It tends to be longer in women under 20 and in women over 40 years of age.

Ovulatory Phase:
Once the dominant follicle has reached its peak hormone levels and growth, a message is sent to the pituitary gland that causes a surge of FSH and another hormone called *lutenizing hormone (LH)*. These hormones cause the follicle to burst, releasing a mature egg, which moves into the open end of the fallopian tube within 2-3 minutes. This is called *ovulation*. It is during this time that a woman is most likely to get pregnant if she and her partner have unprotected intercourse

Menstrual cycle events

[Adapted from: Hatcher RA, et al. *Contraceptive Technology*. 16th ed. New York: Irvington, 1994:41]

Along with each phase in the menstrual cycle, a woman experiences certain physiological changes. Some of the changes occur in all women, while others vary from woman to woman. The figure on this page puts it all together. It shows the different body changes that occur with each phase, including temperature changes, cervical mucus changes, varying hormone levels, and possible menstrual cycle symptoms like mood changes, headaches and cramps. Look vertically to find the point in the menstrual cycle and the possible corresponding events.

Day

1	2	3	4	5	6	7	8	9	10	11	12	13	14	15	16	17	18	19	20	21	22	23	24	25	26	27	28

Phase

Follicular	Luteal

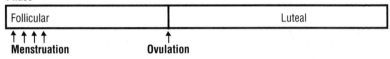

Menstruation   **Ovulation**

Cervical Mucus

Low Volume	High Volume	Low Volume
Thick	Thin	Thick
Cloudy	Clear	Cloudy
Not very stretchy	Very stretchy	Not very stretchy

Basal Body Temperature

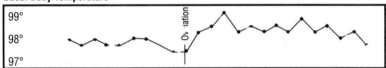

99°
98°
97°

NOTE: example only

Possible Body Changes

Menstrual Phase	Midcycle	Premenstrual Phase
Irritability	Vaginal secretions	Weight gain
Anxiety	Nausea	Bloating
Depression	Sharp or dull pain	Eyes swollen
Bleeding	in the abdomen	Ankles swollen
Lower abdominal pain	Spotting	Breast fullness
Back and leg pain	Increased sex drive	Breast tenderness
Headaches		Anxiety
Nausea		Depression
Dizziness		Headaches
Diarrhea		Nausea
Increased/decreased		Acne
sex drive		Spotting
Infection		Vaginal discharge
Nosebleeds		Pain
		Constipation

Luteal Phase:

Primarily after the egg has been released, the hormone called *progesterone* is produced in a structure called the *corpus luteum*. The corpus luteum is what is left of the ovarian follicle after the egg has been released. Progesterone stops other follicles in the ovaries from growing and helps the lining of the uterus grow in order to prepare for a possible pregnancy. If pregnancy does not occur, the luteal phase tends to be about 14 days long in most women.

Menstruation:

If pregnancy does not occur, the levels of progesterone and estrogen go down during the late luteal phase. This causes the lining of the uterus to stop growing and it is shed, resulting in menstrual bleeding. Most women lose about 30-35 milliliters or about 2 tablespoons of blood during menstruation. It is normal, though, to lose anywhere from 20 to 80 milliliters of blood. Seventy percent of the blood is shed by the second day and 90% by the third day. The average length of the menstrual phase is 4 to 6 days. Bleeding from 2 to 7 days is within normal limits. In general, see your clinician if your periods come more frequently than every 21 days apart or last more than 7 days.

IMPORTANT INFORMATION FOR YOUR HEALTH:

Toxic Shock Syndrome (TSS): TSS is a rare disease caused by some forms of bacteria that are normally found in the vagina of some women. Sometimes, when these bacteria are combined with the use of tampons or contraceptives such as the diaphragm and cervical cap, the risk of TSS increases. Overall, the risk of TSS is low. It has been estimated that each year 1-17 of every 100,000 menstruating women and girls will get TSS. Of the women who have gotten TSS, about 5% have died.

The symptoms of TSS include: a sudden, high fever (usually 102°F or higher); vomiting and/or diarrhea; fainting or near fainting when standing up; dizziness; or a rash that looks like a sunburn. The symptoms of TSS usually appear very quickly and are often severe. Other symptoms may be muscle or joint aches, red eyes, sore throat, and weakness. *If you have any of these symptoms or think you may have TSS, contact your health care provider immediately.*

You can avoid the risk of getting tampon-associated TSS by not using tampons. If you do use tampons, you can reduce your risk of TSS by using the smallest tampon that contains your menstrual flow. You can also lower your risk by sometimes using maxi-pads instead of tampons (such as using pads at night). If you are using a vaginal barrier method, such as the diaphragm or cervical cap, do not keep the barrier in your vagina longer than the recommended time. Know the symptoms of TSS and contact your health care provider immediately if you think you may have TSS.

Douching: Douching is something some women do to clean out the vagina. There are many products sold for this purpose (e.g., Summer's Eve). *However, it is important to know that the vagina is naturally a self-cleaning organ.* Some vaginal discharge and a slight musky odor is *normal*. Using douches, which often contain harsh chemicals, can actually irritate the vagina and trigger infections such as bacterial vaginosis and candidiasis (yeast infections). If you do have abnormal vaginal discharge—heavy or very unusual or bad smelling—it may mean that you have an infection. Contact your health care provider right away.

Let's Talk About Sex!
What Real Couples Have to Say...

"For us, the fundamental basis of our communication about sex is trust and honesty. Even in our most vulnerable moments, we have been open with each other and that has only increased the level of intimacy that we share."

—Tamara, 39 and Keith, 40

"In communicating with a partner about sex, using humor to relieve some of the discomfort and awkwardness works very well. Some advice would be to never take yourself, your partner, or your relationship too seriously and to have fun and be goofy. This will allow open communication about a potentially awkward subject."

—Sammy and Liz, both 27

"Being absolutely honest with my partner makes me feel absolutely secure. The more honest we are, the more connected I feel. My jealousies and insecurities melted away as honesty solidified itself as the foundation of our relationship. If I know her uncensored fantasies and experiences and dreams, I have eliminated one of the most frightening forces in the universe—the unknown. What could be more beautiful than knowing that your partner knows everything about you and accepts you for you?"

—John, 26, on his relationship with Elizabeth, 28

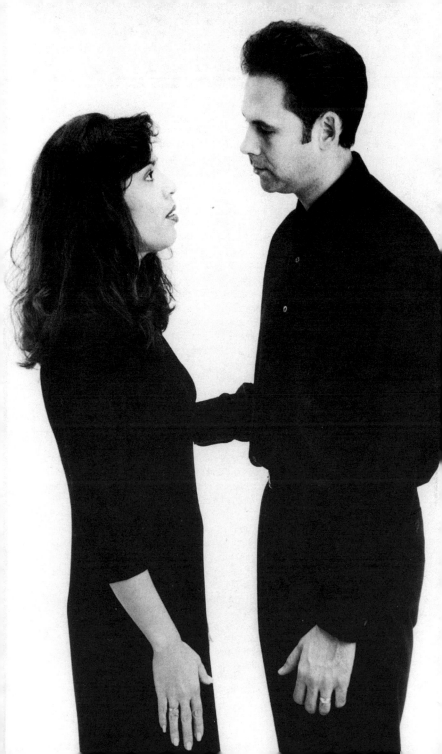

TALKING WITH YOUR PARTNER

Talking to your partner about sexual subjects isn't always the easiest thing to do, but it is important. Sometimes it may seem easier to just have sex rather than talk about it. BUT, there are many important reasons to talk about sex first. Before we get to those reasons, however, let's first look at some of the reasons why it may be hard to talk to your partner about sex:

- No matter what age you are, it is quite possible that nobody taught you how to talk about sex. We learn about many other things in life in a very organized way—how to do math, how to spell, how to drive, how to write a check. But we usually do not learn how to communicate about our sexual body parts, feelings, thoughts, and experiences. So, don't feel alone if you don't know where to start.
- There are some pretty negative stereotypes, or judgments, that go along with people who talk openly about sex. If someone, especially a woman, talks about sex, people may think she is "loose" or "easy." If she does not talk about sex, she may be called a "prude." Often, if it is a guy doing the talking and he is talking in a serious manner about his feelings, his friends may call him a wimp or "too sensitive." Guys that talk about sex in a proud or conquering way may be looked upon as "studs." These stereotypes don't leave a lot of middle ground for healthy communication.
- It is likely that at some point while growing up you learned that sex was a topic to be shy or embarrassed about, even ashamed of. You may have learned names like "wee wee" and "down there" for your sexual body parts, which makes it tough to say "penis" and "clitoris" comfortably to a sex partner. We do not have a good language for sexuality, which is one of the most important things we need in order to communicate.

Now that we've looked at some reasons it may be difficult to talk about sex with a partner, we need to think about why it is so important. Today, more than ever, being honest and open with a sex partner is a health necessity. Because of the risk of sexually transmitted infections (STIs), including HIV/AIDS, you need to be able to have these conversations with a sex partner before you have sex. Asking about your partner's sexual history, whether he or she has had or has been tested for sexually transmitted infections, and what type of protection you will use are all important topics to discuss *before* you hop into bed. Needless to say, bringing these things up in the heat of the moment can ruin the mood! Talking about what, if any, methods of contraception you will use is also important—all a part of having responsible and enjoyable sex. Finally, and most importantly, talking about sex brings you closer to your partner. Increasing intimacy can help connect you, make your relationship stronger, and improve sex.

Because communication is so important, and because we often don't learn how to communicate effectively, especially about sexual topics, we have included some tips on communication skills that will help you and your partner have these conversations.

COMMUNICATION SKILLS

Active Listening: Some people actually say that being able to listen is more important than being able to talk. Certainly it is more difficult for many people. Active listening means that you are paying full attention to your partner—looking him or her in the eye, nodding or shaking your head when he says something, and orienting your body in her direction. Using words and sounds like, "uh huh," "I understand," and "mm hmm" show that you are participating in the conversation. Think about how it feels when you are talking to someone who is not paying attention—looking the other way, looking at the clock, or tapping a pencil. It is quite frustrating. Compare this to how you feel when the other person is looking at you, nodding, and asking you questions. Big difference? That's active listening.

"I" Statements: Using "I" statements is one of the hardest parts of good communication. This means that you are speaking for yourself, owning your statements. Often this means that you are sharing your personal feelings about something. For example, instead of saying, "You never listen to me when I talk to you," you might say, "I feel ignored when I talk to you." When you own what you say, you avoid accusing the other person or making generalizations. "I" statements can also help reduce defensiveness in communication. Doesn't the statement, "For me, oral sex does not feel that good" sound better than the statement, "You know, most women don't like oral sex?"

Self-disclosure: This goes along with using "I" statements. If you are speaking for yourself, you are also sharing, or disclosing, your thoughts and feelings to your partner. Studies have shown that self-disclosure is reciprocal—meaning that the more one partner does it, the more the other partner will. Sharing personal things with your partner, both about sex and about other topics, is one way that the level of intimacy in your relationship will increase.

Paraphrasing: This means saying back to your partner what you thought you heard him or her say. For example, if your partner is angry that you were late and is yelling about how you're never on time, you might say (in a calm voice), "What I hear you saying is that you're really frustrated with me right now because I didn't come home when I said I would." Using a phrase like, "what I hear you saying" or "so, what you mean is" can help make sure you are both on the same page and understanding what's going on in the conversation.

Body Language: Body language, what is sometimes called nonverbal communication, is a huge part of communication. What we do with our bodies while we are talking can support and emphasize what we are saying, or can completely undermine it. For example, if you are saying you feel comfortable talking about sex, but are looking the other direction, tapping your foot, using a soft, mumbling voice, and slouching over, it sends the opposite message to your partner. In some cases, body language can make or break a conversation.

Several Marvelous Quotes from <u>What I've Learned About Sex</u>*:
- Sex is a small part of life, but it becomes very important when it doesn't work out
- It is a myth that sex comes naturally; people need to learn to be good lovers
- Sex is wonderful! You don't have to feel guilty to enjoy it
- Thinking before sex is a good idea; thinking during sex never is
- In some states, it's legal to buy a gun, but not a vibrator

*Haffner, Debra W. and Schwartz, Pepper, *What I've Learned About Sex.* New York, Berkley Publishing Group, 1998

TALKING WITH YOUR HEALTH CARE PROVIDER

Taking Sexual Histories

Talking to a health care provider about sexual subjects and reproductive health can sometimes be challenging and embarrassing. Sometimes it is more embarrassing for the person taking care of you than it is for you. But these conversations may also be critically important in helping you to make good decisions and to maintain health. So, ask your clinician questions if you need help or more information.

It is important to know that in the best-case scenario taking a sexual history is a *routine* part of your clinician's services. All too often it is neglected. It is equally important for you to assess your own sexual history. Below are some *possible* questions that a clinician might ask you and that you can ask *yourself.* If your clinician does not ask you these questions, you can bring up the topic by asking if you are at risk for infections, asking to be tested for infections, asking for information on sexual dysfunction, or other questions like these.

NOTE: You are entitled to confidentiality when discussing all of these issues with your health care provider.

- **What are you doing to protect yourself from HIV and other sexually transmitted infections (STIs)?**
- Have you had a sexual experience with another person in the last year? *If yes, with how many different people?*
- Have your sex partners been men, women, or both?
- How many sex partners have you had, total, in your lifetime?
- Have you had a sexually transmitted infection? *If yes, which infection?*
- Have any of your past partners had an infection that you know of?
- Have you shared needles or injection equipment with any person?
- Have you had intercourse under the influence of drugs, including alcohol?
- Have you awoken and not known whether somebody has had sex with you?
- Has a sexual partner put you at risk of getting an infection?
- What do you do to protect yourself or your partner from pregnancy?
- Has anyone coerced or forced you into having sex with him or her?
- Have you had problems getting aroused or experiencing orgasm?
- Is there anything else about you, as a sexual being, that I should know, so I can provide you with the best possible care?

Advantages of talking openly to your clinician:

- Clear up misinformation and myths—you can get the facts!
- Help you better understand treatments
- Help you change behaviors that are harmful to your health
- Helps you make decisions about contraception and safer sex
- Lets you know of possible side effects
- Lets you know when to return if you need to
- Decreases your risk of serious problems
- Make your relationship with your clinician stronger

Healthy sexual functioning is an important part of your overall health. We have included this brief guide to help you become aware of different sexual problems. If you think one of the descriptions applies to you or your partner, we recommend discussing the issue with your health care provider or a sex counselor or therapist. Most sexual dysfunction can be treated with the help of qualified professionals. To get the number of a certified sex therapist or counselor in your area, contact the American Association of Sex Educators, Counselors, and Therapists (AASECT) by phone at (319) 895-8407 or on the Internet at www.aasect.org.

FEMALE SEXUAL DYSFUNCTION

Decreased Sexual Desire

Decreased sexual desire is when a woman has no or a very low sex drive. This lack of desire is a sexual dysfunction when it causes problems for her personally and in her sexual relationship(s). Decreased desire is relative to a partner's desire. There is no absolute "normal" level. This is a very common problem—about 1 out of every 3 women has a lack of desire for some period of time during her life.

- *What causes it?* The cause is usually psychological. Things like relationship problems, financial stress, and career or school stress might be causing a woman to have less sexual desire. In addition, having been sexually abused in the past, or using drugs and alcohol, can decrease her sexual desire. It can also be related to medical problems like depression, hormone imbalance, and other disorders. For example, having a low level of testosterone may lead to decreased sex drive. Sometimes a woman may have less desire after she starts using a hormonal contraceptive like birth control pills
- *How is it treated?* A woman may need to be examined by a medical doctor and/or a counselor. If a medical problem is causing her to have a lack of desire, that problem can be treated. Sometimes the hormone testosterone is given to increase sex drive. If there are psychological reasons, she and her partner can work with a counselor or therapist to treat the problem. NOTE: If the woman is in a relationship, this is usually *not* "just her problem." It is important that both partners are involved in the treatment. Both partners are affected when one has a lack of sexual desire

Excessive Sexual Desire

Excessive sexual desire is when a woman has sexual desire that is out of her control. It may lead her to act in obsessive-compulsive ways. She may act out her desire in ways that are directly harmful to herself and others (unprotected sex with many partners, child sexual abuse).

- *What causes it?* The causes are complicated. They are usually psychological, related in some way to a woman's past experience. For example, she may have been sexually abused as a child and is acting out what she learned while growing up. Low self-esteem and depression may also be related. Drug or alcohol use can complicate the problem
- *How is it treated?* Treatment varies depending on the type and cause. Individual and group therapy are usually used. Therapeutic techniques used to treat obsessive-compulsive behaviors are often helpful

Anorgasmia: Primary

Primary anorgasmia is when a woman has never had an orgasm—either from masturbating or with a partner.

- *What causes it?* The cause is usually psychological. Some women may not know how their bodies and sexual response cycles work. Others may have performance anxiety— they are so focused on reaching the goal of orgasm (performing) that the anxiety stops them from relaxing enough to do so. Other women may have been taught that sex is bad, or have been abused, which stops them from being able to relax and enjoy sex
- *How is it treated?* Depending on the cause, it is usually treated by seeing a counselor or therapist. There are exercises the couple can do to help decrease the pressure to perform during sex. These are called *sensate focus* exercises, where the woman tries to focus on *all* of her sexual feelings, without trying to achieve the "goal" of orgasm. Getting to know her body through self-pleasuring may also help her identify what feels good to her. If one partner is not able to have an orgasm, this can affect the relationship, so a counselor will most likely want to work with the woman and her partner together

Anorgasmia: Secondary

Secondary anorgasmia is when a woman has had orgasms in the past—either from masturbating or with a partner—but is unable to presently or in certain situations.

- *What causes it?* The cause is usually psychological or situational. For example, a woman may be able to experience orgasm when she masturbates, but not when she is with her partner. (NOTE: If she is able to orgasm during oral sex or mutual masturbation with a partner, but not during intercourse, this does not necessarily mean that she has anorgasmia. *Most* women do not orgasm from penile thrusting alone—stimulation of the clitoris is needed). Other reasons may be having a new partner or having performance anxiety. Medical problems such as neurological (brain, spinal cord, nerves) or vascular (heart, blood vessels) diseases may also cause it. Medicines for depression, blood pressure, and other problems can significantly diminish both sex drive and the ability to have orgasms
- *How is it treated?* Similar treatments are used with secondary anorgasmia as with primary anorgasmia (see above)

Vaginismus

Vaginismus is a painful, spastic contraction (like a cramp) of the pelvic muscles that happens when a woman or man tries to put a penis, finger, or other object into the vagina.

- *What causes it?* The cause is usually psychological. A woman may have been sexually abused, she may be having sex when she does not want to, or she may have been taught that sex is bad or negative. Vaginismus can also happen when sex is painful for a woman due to infection, scarring, or a very small opening of the vagina. Future contractions are then an unconscious response to protect the woman from more pain. NOTE: Sometimes it is difficult to tell the difference between vaginismus and dyspareunia (painful intercourse). It is important to see a qualified health care provider in order to get a correct diagnosis and treatment
- *How is it treated?* It is usually treated using an exercise in which a woman (alone or with her partner) slowly works on relaxing her vagina by inserting progressively larger dilators and consciously relaxing the vaginal muscles

Dyspareunia

Dyspareunia is pain when a penis, finger, or other object is inserted into the vagina.

- *What causes it?* The cause is often related to a medical problem such as a urinary tract infection, a sexually transmitted infection, endometriosis, pelvic inflammatory disease, fibroids, interstitial cystitis, or spinal column disc diseases. Dryness of the vagina may also cause pain. In addition, dyspareunia can be caused by psychological factors such as having been sexually abused, taught that sex is bad, or being in a relationship in which the woman is not happy

- *How is it treated?* It is important to see a qualified health care provider in order to get a correct diagnosis and treatment. Some medical problems, like infections, can be treated to help relieve the pain. Dryness in the vagina can be easily treated using a water-based personal lubricant such as Astroglide. Other medical problems are more difficult to treat and may require the woman and her partner to find sexual positions and activities that are less painful. Seeing a counselor or therapist may be necessary to treat psychological causes and/or to help women and their partners work through the psychological effects of dyspareunia

MALE SEXUAL DYSFUNCTION

Decreased Sexual Desire

Decreased sexual desire is when a man has no or a very low sex drive. This lack of desire is a type of sexual dysfunction when it causes problems for him personally and in his sexual relationship(s). Decreased desire is relative to a partner's desire. There is no absolute "normal" level.

- *What causes it?* The cause is usually psychological. Things like relationship problems, financial stress, and career or school stress might be causing a man to have less sexual desire. In addition, having been sexually abused in the past and using drugs and alcohol can decrease his sexual desire. It can also be related to medical problems like certain diseases, depression, and hormone imbalance. For example, a low level of testosterone may lead to decreased sex drive

- *How is it treated?* A man may need to be examined by a medical doctor and a psychologist. If a medical problem is causing him to have a lack of desire, that problem can be treated. If there are psychological reasons, he and his partner can work with a counselor or therapist to treat the problem. NOTE: If the man is in a relationship, this is not usually "just his problem." It is important that both partners are involved in the treatment. Both partners are affected when one has a lack of sexual desire

---

If you have any questions, ask us at...
www.managingcontraception.com

Excessive Sexual Desire

Excessive sexual desire is when a man has sexual desire that is out of his control. It may lead him to act in obsessive-compulsive ways. He may act out his desire in ways that are directly harmful to others (rape, child sexual abuse, publicly exposing himself, making obscene phone calls).

- *What causes it?* The causes are complicated. They are usually psychological, related in some way to a man's past experience. For example, he may have been sexually abused as a child and is acting out what he learned while growing up. Certain attitudes may also be related, such as believing that women want or deserve to be raped. (NOTE: The act of rape is more about having power and control over the victim than about a sexual turn-on.) Drugs or alcohol frequently complicate the problem
- *How is it treated?* Treatment varies depending on the type and cause. In some cases, a man is jailed for offenses such as rape, incest, and child sexual abuse and will also go through intensive group and individual therapy. Therapeutic techniques used to treat obsessive-compulsive behaviors are often helpful. Medicines such as Depo-Provera are also being given to men to help reduce sexual desire

Early Ejaculation

Early ejaculation is when a man ejaculates (comes) without any voluntary control. It is difficult to say how early is too early. One definition is ejaculation in less than a minute of penile thrusting during sexual intercourse. However, because this can vary greatly for each couple, sex therapists often base the diagnosis on the couple's subjective evaluation of their pleasure and satisfaction rather than on a specific length of time. It is more common among young men.

- *What causes it?* The cause is usually psychological. This is often a learned behavior, which means that a man has formed a "habit" based on his past behavior. For example, boys often learn to masturbate in a setting where they are in a hurry, perhaps trying not to get caught. This habit may then carry over into his sexual behavior with a partner. Rarely, it may also be related to neurological (brain, spinal cord, nerves) diseases such as multiple sclerosis and possibly infections such as urethritis
- *How is it treated?* A man and his partner may work with a counselor to "unlearn" the behavior. There are two techniques that can be used—the "start-stop" technique and the "squeeze" technique. In the "start-stop" technique, the man tells his partner when he is just about to ejaculate. His partner stops stimulating the penis for 30 seconds, then starts again. In the "squeeze" technique, the man tells his partner when he is just about to ejaculate. His partner gently squeezes below the glans (head) of the penis for 4-5 seconds. Both techniques can be repeated during sexual activity until the man has more control over his ejaculation. Finally, using condoms or taking small doses of the anti-depressant Prozac might also help treat early ejaculation

Delayed Ejaculation

Delayed ejaculation is when a man is unable to or has problems having an orgasm during sexual activity with a partner.

- *What causes it?* Similar to early ejaculation, the cause is usually psychological and often reflects a learned behavior. For example, a man may masturbate in a way that allows him to orgasm. When he cannot repeat this pattern with a partner, he may have trouble having an orgasm. It may also happen if a man has performance anxiety, that is, feels so much pressure to orgasm that it gets in the way of him doing so. Finally, it is important that a man get checked by a health care provider to make sure that medical problems are not the cause

- *How is it treated?* Some sex therapists use what is called a "demand" strategy, in which a man's partner stimulates his penis manually and switches to intercourse just as he is about to orgasm. Other experts prefer to treat delayed ejaculation similar to anorgasmia in a woman. In this method, called "sensate focus," the couple tries to take the pressure to ejaculate off of the man by having him focus on *all* sexual feelings rather than just trying to reach the "goal" of orgasm. This way, the couple is not trying to *force* the man to have an orgasm

Erectile Dysfunction: Primary
Primary erectile dysfunction (ED) is when a man has never been able to get an erection that allows him to have sexual intercourse. This is an uncommon problem that usually occurs when a man has high levels of anxiety about sexual performance. It is a good idea for a man to have medical and psychological exams to determine the cause and best treatment.

Erectile Dysfunction: Secondary
Secondary erectile dysfunction (ED) is when a man has been able to get erections in the past and cannot currently, or can get an erection in some situations (masturbation) but not in others (with a partner). This is a common problem. About 30 million men in the US have ED, and half of those are under age 65. A man is more likely to have ED as he gets older: about 1 in 20 men 40 years or older and about 1 in 4 men 65 years or older.
- *What causes it?* In the past, it was thought that ED was "all in a man's head" but we now know that this is not the case. In fact, approximately 85% of men with ED have a physical cause for the problem. Diabetes is the most common cause (about 50-60% of men with diabetes have erectile dysfunction). Other causes include heart disease, spinal cord injury, using alcohol, cigarettes, or other drugs, and taking certain prescription medicines such as antidepressants
- *How is it treated?* A man needs to have a medical exam to determine if a physical factor is the cause. If it is physical, there are many medical treatments available (see special section on Viagra and Viagra alternatives). Counseling may be needed for psychological causes or if erectile dysfunction has caused problems in a man's relationship.

SPECIAL SECTION: VIAGRA (SILDENAFIL) AND ALTERNATIVES
Because Viagra is one of the most popular drugs in the United States, we have included some details on the use of this drug and on other treatments for erectile dysfunction. In addition, it can be dangerous, even fatal, when combined with certain commonly used medicines. Thus, we have included important information on dangerous combinations for your safety. Go to www.viagra.com for more information about Viagra.

The following information is adapted from the Viagra package insert:

What is Viagra?
- A treatment for erectile dysfunction. It is a tablet that contains a citrate salt of sildenafil. Sildenafil citrate helps relax the smooth muscles in the penis, allowing blood to flow into the penis which causes an erection when there is sexual stimulation. The tablets are taken by mouth before sexual activity
- Viagra comes in blue, rounded, diamond-shaped tablets. It is available in 25 milligrams, 50 milligrams and 100 milligrams

How effective is Viagra?
- In clinical studies with people who had varying degrees of erectile dysfunction, 63%, 74%, and 82% of men on 25 milligrams, 50 milligrams and 100 milligrams of Viagra, respectively, reported an improvement in their erections, compared to 24% on placebo pills.
  NOTE: Physical and/or visual stimulation is needed to experience erection

Who cannot take Viagra?
- People who may be hypersensitive to a part of the tablet, such as people taking organic nitrates, should not take Viagra. Organic nitrates are often taken to prevent heart attacks. They are also found in some drugs used to treat yeast infections and in illegal drugs such as "poppers" (amyl nitrate). If you are taking an organic nitrate, you should NOT take Viagra. See the warning box below for a list of drugs that should not be mixed with Viagra. **Always check with your clinician or pharmacist before mixing any drugs**

What are the possible side effects?
- Taking certain drug combinations with Viagra can be dangerous. Viagra should NOT be taken by people taking nitrates in any form because the combination of the two drugs can severely decrease blood pressure
- There is a potential risk of heart attack during sexual activity in men with pre-existing heart disease. Therefore, treatments for erectile dysfunction, including Viagra, should be used only after careful discussion with a qualified medical professional in men for whom sexual activity is inadvisable because of their underlying heart problem
- *Other side effects are:* headaches (16%), flushing (10%), upset stomach (7%), nasal congestion (4%), UTI (3%), abnormal vision (3%), diarrhea (3%), dizziness (2%), and rash (2%). The abnormal vision in which the colors blue and green may be confused could be hazardous for pilots

How much is taken and how often?
- The usual recommended dose is 50 milligrams taken by mouth, as needed, approximately 1 hour before sexual activity. Based on effectiveness and tolerance, the dose may be increased to the maximum recommended dose of 100 milligrams or decreased to 25 milligrams. The maximum recommended dosing frequency is once per day.

Can women take Viagra?
- Viagra is not approved for use by women. Currently, Viagra use in women is being studied. Some researchers have found a moderate increase in blood flow to the pelvic area and an increase in vaginal lubrication. Others have not found significant effects. However, as of now, side effects are not fully understood

---

Warning: These organic nitrates can be fatal to a person who is taking Viagra

Nitroglycerin	Nitropress	**Isosorbide Mononitrate**	**Pentaerythritol Tetranitrate**
Deponit	Nitroglycerin	Imdur	Peritrate
Nitroprex	Minitran	ISMO	Peritrate SA
Nitro SA	Nitroglycerin T/R	Isosorbide Mononitrate	
Nitrek	Nitroglyn	Monoket	**Erythrityl Tetranitrate**
Nitrospan	Nitro-Bid		Cardilate
Nitrostat	Nitrolingual Spray	**Isosorbide Nitrate**	
Nitrocine	Nitrolan	Dilatrate-SR	**Isosorbide Dinitrate/**
Nitro-Derm	Nitro-Trans System	Isordil Tembids	**Phenobarbital**
Nitro Disc	Nitrol Ointment	Sorbitrate	Isordil w/PB
Nitrong	Nitro Transdermal	Iso-Bid	
Nitro-Time	Nitro-Dur	Sorbitate SA	
Nitropar	Transderm-Nitro	Isosorbide Dinitrate Isordil	
Nitrogard	Tridil	Isosorbide	
		Dinitrate LA	

DANGER: *Examples of dangerous combinations with Viagra*

1. A man is taking organic nitrates to prevent a heart attack. Without knowing the risk, he also takes Viagra. Both of these drugs cause his blood pressure to go down when taken alone. When he takes them together, his blood pressure drops severely and he has to be rushed to the hospital.

2. A woman is being treated for a yeast infection with a drug that contains an organic nitrate (e.g. Diflucan). Her husband is taking Viagra and it has worked wonders for their sexual relationship. She is curious about how it might help her, so she takes one of his tablets. Soon after, her blood pressure drops severely and she goes into shock.

3. A teenage boy often goes out to dance clubs with his friends. Sometimes they take "poppers" (amyl nitrate) when they go, and they have tonight. When he comes home, he is still fairly high and his friends dare him to take one of his father's Viagra tablets that they found in the bathroom. He does and in the next couple of hours begins to have trouble breathing. It gets so bad that he passes out and his friends call 911.

ALTERNATIVE TREATMENTS FOR ERECTILE DYSFUNCTION

Vacuum Erection Device (VED)
- Use of a vacuum pump and different size elastic bands help a man get and keep an erection for 30 minutes by drawing blood into the penis. This method is safe and effective and has up to a 90% success rate. It may be hard to use for some men and may decrease the spontaneity of sexual activity. It may be ideal for others

Urethral Insert
- A small pellet is inserted into the penis which contains prostaglandin E[1] (alprostadil). This causes an erection when it's absorbed into the tissue. Drawbacks include: must be inserted into the penis, expense (cost for one use about $25 to $30 depending on the strength of the dose), mild penile pain in some men. It has about a 70% success rate

Injection Therapy
- A man injects Prostaglandin E[1] (alprostadil) into the spongy tissue of the penis. Erection lasts 30 - 60 minutes and stimulation is necessary. Most men do not mind the minor discomfort of the injection. Priapism (painful, long-lasting erection) can be a problem if too much of the drug is injected (this can be dangerous but it only occurs in 0.5% of all men)

Yohimbine hydrochloride
- A prescription drug made of indole alkaloid (initially taken from the bark of the yohimbehe tree). It is taken by mouth. Recent studies show modest effectiveness but experts believe much of the effect may be placebo, meaning that the drug does not really help a man get an erection. Side effects are minimal, but it does cause increased anxiety and hallucinations in people with psychosis

Penile Implants (Prostheses)
- Bendable rods or inflatable reservoirs are permanently implanted into penis. Success is high, but natural erections may never return

Microsurgery
- Used in men with problems in the penile arteries or veins. It has over a 50% success rate

Forty-eight percent of all U.S. teens between the ages of 13 and 18 have had sexual intercourse—nearly 70% by the age of 18. The authors believe that abstinence from sexual intercourse (oral, vaginal and anal) is best for individuals who are not ready to have responsible sex. However, we also believe that anyone who engages in sexual intercourse should have knowledge about and access to contraception, protection against sexually transmitted infections, and reproductive health services.

It is important for teens to have an open dialogue with a trusted adult, such as a parent, teacher, or health care provider. It is normal to feel embarrassed or shy, but talking to an adult can help teens dispel myths, answer questions, and get advice. For related information on teen health, see: www.advocatesforyouth.org.

Misconceptions: It is common for young people to have misconceptions about pregnancy. In fact, chances are many adults have incorrect information, too. So, pay close attention to this section. You may learn something new that you can teach someone else.

MYTH: *"You cannot get pregnant the first time you have intercourse."*
FACT: Conception can occur at first intercourse, even before periods begin.

MYTH: *"You cannot get pregnant without penetration."*
FACT: Seminal fluid introduced outside the vagina can enter the vagina and cause pregnancy.

MYTH: *"If you have not had a period, you cannot become pregnant."*
FACT: Ovulation (see pages 5-6) can occur before a girl starts having periods, making pregnancy possible.

MYTH: *"You cannot get pregnant if you douche after sex."*
FACT: Douching does not remove or kill all semen; it is still possible to get pregnant.

Confidentiality: It's natural to be concerned about confidentiality. The authors believe that all teens should be able to get confidential services and counseling but laws exist in some states that restrict teen access to family planning services. To help you understand these laws, we have included this table, which provides information on the rights teens have to consent to reproductive health, contraception and abortion services.

WHAT ARE YOUR STATE'S LAWS FOR TEEN REPRODUCTIVE HEALTH SERVICES?

AL ●■	FL ◆*	LA ●■	NE ●*	OK ◆	VT ●
AK ◆■	GA ◆*	ME ◆	NV ●*	OR ◆	VA ◆*
AZ ●■	HI ◆	MD ◆*	NH ●	PA ●■	WA ●
AR ◆*	ID ◆■	MA ●■	NJ ●*	RI ●■	WV ●*
CA ◆■	IL ◆*	MN ●*	NM ◆■	SC ●■	WI ●■
CO ◆*	IN ●■	MI ●■	NY ◆	SD ●*	WY ◆■
CT ●	IA ●*	MS ◆■	NC ◆■	TN ◆■	
DE ◆*	KS ●*	MO ●■	ND ●■	TX ●*	
DC ◆	KY ◆■	MT ◆*	OH ●*	UT ●*	

◆ = States where minors (under 18 years) can receive reproductive health care including treatment of STIs and contraception without parental notification or consent (as of 10/97)

● = No consent laws exist for minors seeking reproductive health care and contraception (as of 10/97)

■ = States with mandatory parental consent laws for minors seeking abortions (as of 2/00)

* = States requiring *parental notification*, but not *parental consent*. *Consent* means a parent must be present during the abortion. *Notification* means the minor must provide a signed statement from the parent(s) stating that the parent has been notified that an abortion is to be performed on the minor

* *Issues in Brief*, "Teenagers Right to Consent to Reproductive Health Care," The Alan Guttmacher Institute, 1997.
Facts in Brief, "Teen Sex and Pregnancy," The Alan Guttmacher Institute, 1997.
The Status of Major Abortion-Related Laws and Policies in the States, Alan Guttmacher Institute, February, 2000.
(Laws in effect as of July, 2000)

WHAT IS MENOPAUSE?

The point at which a woman permanently stops having monthly periods following the decline of estrogen production in the ovaries. *Perimenopause* is the period leading up to menopause, when a woman may experience some of the physical changes that go along with menopause. See www.menopause.org for related information.

Average age of perimenopause (irregular periods): 46 years old
Average age of menopause: 51 years old

Common physical changes:
- Hot flashes
- Mood changes
- Thinning of the walls of the vagina
- Vaginal dryness
- Loss of calcium from the bones
- Increased likelihood of *atherogenesis* (the formation of fat deposits in the arteries which leave a woman at risk of heart attack and stroke)

WHAT ABOUT CONTRACEPTION DURING PERIMENOPAUSE?

- It is important to remember that even with decreasing fertility a woman needs contraception until menopause if she does not want to become pregnant. Up to 75% of pregnancies in women over 40 are unintended
- All currently available contraceptives can be used until menopause
- Pills are ideal for the healthy, non-smoking woman who has irregular periods during perimenopause since they regulate cycles and maintain estrogen levels
- Long-acting methods like the IUD and Norplant are an excellent way to have a single decision provide long-term contraception until menopause
- Sterilization is popular in this age group. Fifty percent of all women ages 40-44 who practice contraception have been sterilized and another 20% have a male partner with a vasectomy

WHAT IS HORMONE REPLACEMENT THERAPY (HRT)?

HRT involves taking hormones—estrogen and, if the woman still has a uterus, progestin— to supplement decreasing hormone levels that occur when a woman begins approaching menopause. HRT may help relieve some of the symptoms of menopause such as hot flashes, vaginal thinning, and mood changes and can help prevent osteoporosis (bone thinning) and cardiovascular disease. It may also help prevent Alzheimer's disease, colon cancer, and tooth loss. Your clinician should advise you of all the risks and benefits of HRT. The decision to begin HRT is complex and must be carefully reviewed by the woman with her health care provider.

WHAT IS INVOLVED IN TAKING HRT?

- Your clinician should take a general medical history and do a physical exam (including a breast and pelvic exam). She or he will take your blood pressure, do a Pap smear, may check your blood lipid profile (e.g., cholesterol), and do a mammogram
- If you have had a hysterectomy (removal of the uterus), you will probably be given estrogen alone
- If you have a uterus, you will receive a progestin with the estrogen to prevent endometrial (uterine) cancer
- You will probably take estrogen continuously (i.e., a daily pill or as a patch); you can also take estrogen vaginally in the form of creams or rings
- You will take progestin in a cyclic fashion (e.g., a pill for 12-14 days a month, which results in a monthly bleed when you stop taking the pill) or continuously (daily) in a lower dose pill; you can also take progestin vaginally in the form of a gel
- Combination estrogen/progestin medicines are available (e.g., Prempro, Premphase, Combipatch)
- Combination estrogen/testosterone medicines are also available (Estratest). For some women, the hormone testosterone helps increase sexual desire

WHAT ARE THE ADVANTAGES OF HRT?

- Helps relieve some of the symptoms of perimenopause: hot flashes, mood changes, irregular periods, and thinning of the vaginal walls
- Prevents osteoporosis and heart disease
- May help prevent Alzheimer's disease, colon cancer, and tooth decay
- When estrogen and progestin are taken together, the combination may decrease the risk of uterine cancer
- When HRT is taken at night, it may help women with sleep disturbance

WHAT ARE THE DISADVANTAGES OF HRT?

- Side effects may include breast tenderness, breast engorgement, vaginal bleeding/spotting, nausea, bloating
- If estrogen is taken alone by a woman who still has her uterus, there is an increased risk of uterine cancer. When estrogen is taken with progestin, the risk of uterine cancer is the same or lower compared to women not taking HRT
- Research results conflict about the risk of breast cancer when taking HRT. Some studies show an increased risk if estrogen is taken alone, while others do not. Similarly, some show a decreased risk of breast cancer if estrogen is taken with progestin, while others show no difference. Continuing concern and awareness need to be shown until the relationship between HRT and breast cancer is better understood. All women in this age group should have regular mammograms and should do monthly breast self exams (BSE)
- It is recommended that women who have had breast cancer not take HRT; however, recently, small studies show no increase in risk of breast cancer returning

The First Step in Planning a Family...

...begins with the decision to become pregnant and bear a child. This active decision-making process should include a commitment by both partners to participate in the love, care, education and financial support of that miraculous child which will result from a few minutes of sexual intercourse. This is a very long-term commitment.

Family planning includes the prepregnancy considerations discussed in this chapter including taking folic acid (at least 0.4 milligrams daily) in advance of pregnancy; deciding to stop smoking or drinking alcohol or taking other drugs during pregnancy; preventing and testing for sexually transmitted infections which might affect the baby; and choosing who will care for you medically during your pregnancy.

The family to the right is among the many, many planned families. When the first U.S. Census was done the average woman had 8 children and methods of birth control were limited. Today, the average woman has approximately 2 children. Advanced contraceptive technology and medical knowledge give men and women many options to control fertility and help them have healthy pregnancies. Safe, effective contraception and knowledge of what to do to have healthy pregnancies are important to the health of mothers, babies, and families.

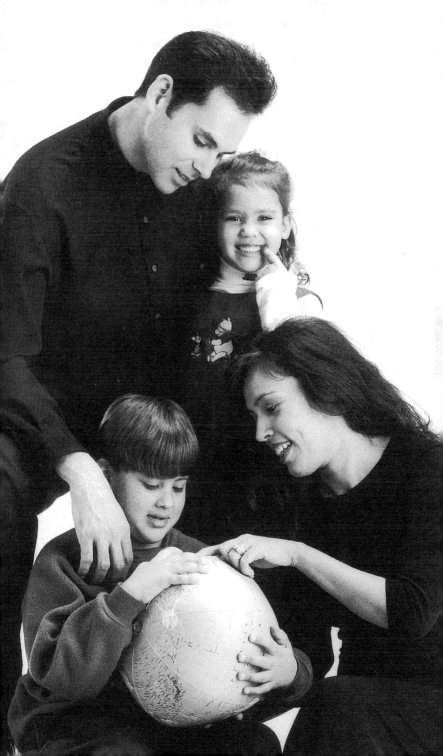

Actively choosing to become pregnant is a very important decision—perhaps one of the most important decisions you will make during your life. In creating a new life, it is critical to remember that the developing fetus is affected by everything the pregnant mother does, including: eating, physical activity, sleeping, and harmful things such as smoking, drinking, and doing drugs. Some things the mother can control, such as taking a daily vitamin with 0.4 mg of folic acid and all other substances she chooses to put into her body. Some things she cannot control, such as a family history of certain illnesses or genetic problems. Other things may or may not be in her control, such as environmental factors such as where she lives and works. In all circumstances, if you are considering becoming pregnant, it is important to ask yourself the following questions and *to discuss each of them with a health care provider:*

Do you:
____ Smoke? **(If yes, it is very important that you quit while you are pregnant)**
____ Use alcohol? **(You should not drink during pregnancy. Even small amounts of alcohol can cause problems with a baby's development)**
____ Use illegal drugs? **(If yes, you need to stop to protect the health of the baby and your own health)**
____ Have good nutrition habits?
____ Live near or work in conditions that may pose risks to pregnancy (strenuous physical work, chemicals, radiation, etc.)?
____ Take any medicines that may be harmful? (Be sure to discuss all medicines, including vitamins, or herbs, you take with your clinician. Do not stop or start taking any without talking to your clinician first)

Have you been tested or examined for:
____ Human immunodeficiency virus (HIV)?
____ Syphilis?
____ Hepatitis B or C?
____ Tuberculosis (TB)?
____ Chlamydia, gonorrhea, herpes, human papilloma virus (HPV)?

Have you had:
____ Rubella immunization? (If not, you should wait 3 months after you get it before you try to get pregnant)
____ Chicken pox? (If not, you should be tested and receive a vaccine if you are not immune)
____ Tetanus immunization? (If not, you should receive an immunization)
____ Pap test? (If not, it is very important to get one as part of a prepregnancy check-up)

Have you talked to a	____	Sickle-cell anemia?
clinician if you have	____	Tay-Sachs, Canavan disease?
a family history of:	____	Previous pregnancy problems such as mental retardation or birth defects?
	____	Alpha or beta-Thalassemia?
	____	Cystic fibrosis?
	____	Seizure disorder?
	____	Diabetes?
Do you live near or	____	Pesticides?
work with:	____	Lead or mercury?
Are you experiencing	____	Domestic violence?
(or have you	____	Emotional or relationship problems?
experienced):	____	Depression?
	____	Financial problems?
Recommended:	____	Protect yourself from STIs (always use a condom if you are at risk of getting an infection during pregnancy)
	____	Eat a healthy diet (talk to your clinician about the best diet for you)
	____	**Take a vitamin with at least 0.4 mg folic acid per day**
	____	Use gloves for outdoor gardening
	____	Lose weight if you are overweight
	____	Get moderate exercise (talk to your clinician about the best exercise plan for you)
Avoid these:	____	Raw meat or fish
	____	Unpasteurized dairy products
	____	Abdominal X-rays, unless necessary
	____	Excessive vitamin intake
	____	Raising body temperature (such as in a jacuzzi)
	____	Getting a new cat (cat feces can be dangerous to pregnant women)
	____	Excessive exercise
Choosing a clinician:	____	Planning a pregnancy also involves trusting the health care provider that will care for you during your pregnancy and birth. Knowing this person before pregnancy creates a smooth transition to pre- and postnatal care. The following websites have information about finding the clinician best for you:

• www.acog.org (American College of Obstetrics & Gynecology)
• www.acnm.org (American College of Nurse-Midwives)
• www.aafp.org (American Academy of Family Physicians)

CHAPTER 9

Pregnancy Testing

WHAT ARE PREGNANCY TESTS AND WHY ARE THEY IMPORTANT?

- Clinical tests look for the hormone called human chorionic gonadotropin (HCG) in the urine and are complete in 1-5 minutes
- Clinical urine pregnancy tests are positive when HCG levels reach 25 or more. By the time a woman realizes that she is missing her menstrual period and suspects she is pregnant, her HCG level will be in the range of 50 to 250. This means that a sensitive urine pregnancy test, one that is done in your clinician's office, may actually be positive **before** a woman misses her period
- You can also use home tests, but they may be misinterpreted. **Therefore, it is important to see a health care provider to confirm your pregnancy**
- Early testing can give you a head start on prenatal care or make it possible for you to get a medical abortion (before you are 3 months (12 weeks) pregnant)
- If you are at risk for ectopic pregnancy (a pregnancy outside of the uterus, usually in the fallopian tubes) because you have had a sexually transmitted infection, disease of the fallopian tubes, pelvic surgery, endometriosis, or an ectopic pregnancy in the past, you should be tested and counseled early. HCG test on a woman's blood are used in the evaluation of a woman for an ectopic pregnancy. Early management of an ectopic pregnancy has saved many women's lives and has preserved many women's fallopian tubes

WHAT IS HCG?

- Human chorionic gonadotropin (HCG) is a hormone produced by the developing placenta (the organ that joins the mother and the fetus) and by the fertilized egg after it implants in the uterus. HCG helps maintain the pregnancy
- HCG is the hormone that is used to detect pregnancy in urine and blood tests

WHAT IF THE PREGNANCY TEST IS POSITIVE?

If your pregnancy test is positive, it is important to be aware of your options. Talking with someone you trust (a family member, your partner, a minister, rabbi, or priest, or a health care provider) may help you make a decision. Your pregnancy options include:

- Carry the pregnancy to term, give birth, and keep child. If this is the option you choose, it is important that you go to a health care provider for prenatal care as soon as possible. Start taking 0.4 mg of folic acid every day. STOP drinking, smoking, or taking other drugs
- Carry the pregnancy to term, give birth, and place the child up for adoption. Again, if this is the option you choose, it is important that you go to a health care provider for prenatal care as soon as possible
- End the pregnancy by getting an abortion. If this is your decision, it is important to know that abortion is a safe, legal, and effective procedure that is best performed early in the pregnancy. Therefore, you need to see a health care provider as soon as possible. (For more information on abortion, see chapter 11)

While you are pregnant, it is important to think about the contraceptive method you will use after you give birth. There are specific considerations about when and how to start different methods because of the changes a woman's body experiences during pregnancy and because she may or may not be breastfeeding.

WHAT ARE MY CONTRACEPTIVE OPTIONS AFTER BIRTH?

Before I leave the hospital:

- You can start breastfeeding and that act alone, under specific conditions, can be used as a contraceptive method (see page 42)
- Combined oral contraceptive pills (COCs) may be prescribed or provided to you. You can start pills 21 days after birth or the Sunday thereafter (if you are **not** breast feeding)
- Progestin-only pills (POPs) may be prescribed or provided to you and it is possible to start them when you leave the hospital (whether or not you are nursing) (there is some concern if you have had gestational diabetes; see page 92)
- Norplant implants may be inserted (whether or not you are nursing)
- IUD may be inserted (whether or not you are nursing) if the necessary instruments are available
- Condoms can be used and can help prevent against infection—women who have just given birth are at a greater risk for pelvic infection than at any other time in their life
- Tubal sterilization may be performed, either during a cesarian section or as a separate procedure 12-48 hours after delivery
- Depo-Provera may be given (whether or not you are nursing)

At my office visit about 4-6 weeks after giving birth:

- If breastfeeding, you should strongly consider using a back-up method of contraception, and you should definitely not count on breastfeeding as your contraceptive if you are giving your baby supplemental feedings with formula or food, if your periods have returned, or if you are breastfeeding infrequently (see page 42)
- If you are not breastfeeding, you should wait until your baby is 3 weeks old to start taking combined pills.
- If you are nursing and combined pills are the only method you will consider, you should wait until your baby is 6 weeks old before you start pills. Use condoms until you start pills and for the first 7 days of pill use
- Other combined hormonal methods may be started 3 weeks after you give birth
- Progestin-only pills (POPs) may be started right away (whether or not you are nursing)
- Norplant implants may be inserted (whether or not you are nursing)
- IUD may be inserted (whether or not you are nursing)
- Condoms can be used as a primary method or as back-up; they can help prevent against infection
- Tubal sterilization may be scheduled (or a vasectomy for a male partner)
- Depo-Provera injection may be given (whether or not you are nursing)
- Diaphragm or cervical cap may be fitted if it does not cause pain in or around the vagina (wait if you are still healing from an episiotomy or tearing)
- You can take emergency contraception if you need it (whether or not you are nursing)

"My period is late and my pregnancy test is positive!"

It's an emotionally-charged moment when a woman is late for her period and is aware that she may be pregnant. She may have been hoping to become pregnant for months or years. She may not want to be pregnant at the present time. Usually, of course, this knowledge of her pregnancy is shared by a woman with her husband or partner. His responses may be as varied as the responses she might have.

In the United States, just over half of women who find that they are pregnant go on to give birth. From 10-20% have a spontaneous miscarriage (a spontaneous abortion) after the diagnosis of a pregnancy is made. The remaining women choose to have a pregnancy termination procedure done—an abortion. If an abortion is performed early in pregnancy under safe conditions it is extremely safe. In fact, very early abortions are slightly safer than carrying a pregnancy to term. When abortions are difficult for women to obtain, done late in pregnancy, or done under unsafe conditions, they become more dangerous. The complications of unsafe abortions are a leading cause of maternal mortality throughout the world.

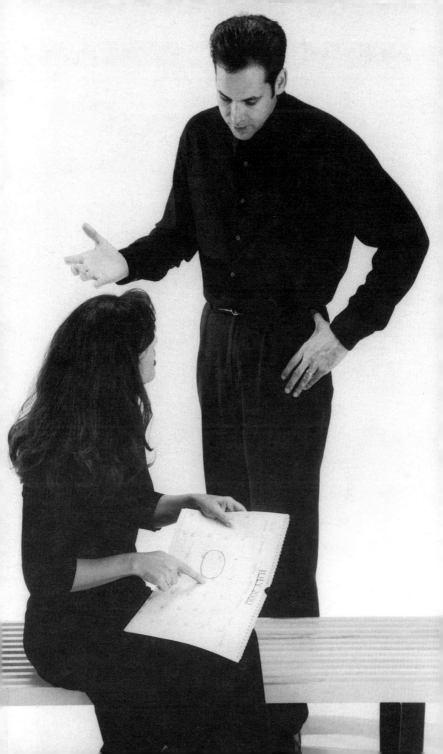

PREGNANCY TERMINATION: SURGICAL ABORTION

WHAT IS A SURGICAL ABORTION?

In 1973, the landmark supreme court case, Roe v. Wade, legalized the option of abortion for all women in the U.S. Surgical abortion is voluntary termination of pregnancy using the surgical technique called suction curettage. In a surgical abortion, instruments are used to remove the pregnancy from the uterus. Right now, about 50% of pregnancies are unintended and about 43% of these end in abortion. About 88% of abortions are first-trimester (first 12 weeks) and 97% use suction curettage.

Abortion is a controversial issue in the U.S. and laws change frequently. For current information on your state's abortion laws, contact the National Abortion Rights Action League (202-973-3000; www.naral.org) for a copy of "A State-by-State Review of Abortion and Reproductive Rights."

HOW EFFECTIVE IS A SURGICAL ABORTION?

• More than 99% effective for pregnancies in the uterus

WHAT ACTUALLY HAPPENS DURING A SURGICAL ABORTION?

• Anesthesia is given; it is usually local (numbing the area) rather than general (being put to sleep)
• The cervix (the opening to the uterus) may be opened in advance using special substances
• Using sterile techniques, a suction-tipped plastic tube is inserted into the uterus and contents of uterus are removed through tube
• Usually the uterine cavity is explored with a special instrument to confirm that the abortion is complete

HOW MUCH DOES A SURGICAL ABORTION COST?

Timing	Managed-Care Setting	Public-Provider Setting
Before 12 weeks	highly variable	$130 - 310
12-26 weeks	highly variable	$1800 - 2000

WHAT ARE THE ADVANTAGES OF A SURGICAL ABORTION?

• Provides women with reproductive choice—the ability to prevent an unintended birth or an infant with birth defects
• Safe method when performed under proper conditions by a qualified professional
• Exam and procedure may be done in single visit (NOTE: local laws may affect this)
• Can be performed safely and effectively through second trimester (24 weeks)
• No increased risk of infertility, cervical problems, early labor, birth defects, or breast cancer after an initial first-trimester abortion*[Hogue, 1982]*
• Statistically safer than continuing pregnancy. If performed in the first trimester there is less than 1 death per 100,000 abortions compared to about 9 deaths per 100,000 births *[Hakin, Elahi 1990]*

WHAT ARE THE DISADVANTAGES OF SURGICAL ABORTION?

• If a woman gets an infection after an abortion, there may be related problems such as increased risk of fallopian tube infection, ectopic pregnancy or infertility
• Can be painful if woman is awake
• Every woman must weigh the possibility of regret from having an abortion against the problems that might occur (physically & emotionally) by carrying the pregnancy to term
• May face protesters at some abortion clinics

25

WHAT ARE THE RISKS OF SURGICAL ABORTION?

Infection	up to 3%
Incomplete abortion	0.5%-1.0%
Bleeding	.03%-1.0%
Blood clots in uterus	less than 1%
Failed abortion	0.1%-0.5%
Perforated uterus	0.1%
Death	less than 1 per 100,000 abortions

WHO CAN HAVE A SURGICAL ABORTION?

- Anyone with an unintended pregnancy who wants or needs to end the pregnancy within 20 weeks of conception (the earlier the better)
- Anyone who has given fully informed consent. All aspects of the procedure, the risks of the procedure and the alternatives to the procedure should be explained and a consent form must be signed

What About Adolescents? State laws differ (see page 18). Rates of abortion are higher due to high number of unintended pregnancies among adolescents.

WHAT SHOULD I DO BEFORE A SURGICAL ABORTION?

- Consider and discuss alternatives with your partner, a friend, family member, or health care provider. Your clinician will have referrals for adoption and prenatal care if you choose one of these options
- You will need to find a clinic that will perform the abortion
- You will need to sign an informed consent form
- You should receive emotional support, education, and pre- and post-abortion instructions from a clinician
- Except for women with severe heart or lung disease, blood clots, severe anemia (low blood count), mental disorders, severe fear of pain, or pregnancy beyond 12-14 weeks, abortions can be performed in an outpatient clinic with local anesthesia
- You may want to have your partner, a friend, or family member go with you to the clinic
- Consider contraceptive methods and obtain needed medicines or supplies to avoid another unintended pregnancy

WHAT SHOULD I DO AFTER A SURGICAL ABORTION?

- Have a 24-hour telephone number available for emergencies
- You may want to have your partner, a friend, or family member drive you home or help you get transportation
- Rest for 24 hours after the abortion
- Avoid heavy lifting or straining for 1-2 days
- You may return to work after 24 hours if you feel that you are able
- Bleeding or spotting with some mild cramping is possible in the first week after the procedure and should improve with time
- Use a pain reliever such as ibuprofen or Tylenol for cramping
- Avoid tampon use; change pads often
- No sexual intercourse or douching for 2 weeks
- Take all medicines as directed
- Showers, baths, and swimming are OK
- Arrange an appointment with your clinician to discuss how to avoid future unintended pregnancies

CONTACT YOUR CLINICIAN IF:

• You have a temperature above 100.4°
• Your bleeding pattern is excessive (more than 4 pads get filled with blood in 2 hours)
• You have any severe abdominal pain
• You experience any mood changes, depression or guilty feelings

WHAT HAPPENS IF:

I get an infection? Your clinician should be alerted. She or he will likely treat the infection with antibiotics at the time of an exam. Infection can be avoided at the time of abortion or afterwards by taking prohylactic (preventative) antibiotics.

I bleed? Some bleeding is expected. It should not be more than your normal period. Contact your clinician if you are concerned.

The abortion fails? This is rare but it can happen. You would have symptoms of ongoing pregnancy—missed periods, morning sickness, enlarged uterus. Your clinician should make sure you do not have an ectopic pregnancy, do an ultrasound and then repeat the abortion procedure if necessary.

The abortion is incomplete? You might have cramping and bleeding. The abortion must be repeated.

PREGNANCY TERMINATION:
MEDICAL ABORTION WITH METHOTREXATE (MTX)

WHAT IS MEDICAL ABORTION WITH MTX?

Medical abortion uses a chemical called methotrexate. Given as an injection or orally, methotrexate blocks the hormone that helps the embryo to grow. This ends the pregnancy.

HOW EFFECTIVE IS A MEDICAL ABORTION WITH MTX?

Approximately 90% of abortions are complete if performed before 49 days have passed since the first day of your last menstrual period.

HOW DOES MEDICAL ABORTION WITH MTX WORK?

It chemically interferes with the process that causes cells to grow in the embryo and also prevents growth of the placenta. Often, clinicians use misopristol with methotrexate. Misopristol causes uterine contractions, which expel the embryo.

HOW MUCH DOES MEDICAL ABORTION WITH MTX COST?

Injection MTX + misoprostol: $30
Oral MTX + misoprostol: $23
Actual costs will also include the price of office visits.

IN WHAT WAYS IS MEDICAL ABORTION WITH MTX BETTER THAN SURGICAL ABORTION?

• Very early abortions can be performed
• Private method
• Can be used for ectopic pregnancy (when the egg implants outside of the uterus)
• Less risk of cervical or uterine injury than with surgical procedure
• Probably less risk of infection or hemorrhage
• Some women feel more in control of the abortion procedure or feel it is more "natural"
• Avoids the use of anesthesia

WHAT ARE THE DISADVANTAGES OF MEDICAL ABORTION WITH MTX?

- Cramping, abdominal pain, bleeding, nausea, vomiting, diarrhea, headache, and mouth irritation can occur
- In rare cases, hair loss or low white blood cell count
- Bleeding and the abortion process can last up to several weeks in some women
- MTX and misoprostol are harmful to a developing fetus. **Follow-up is necessary** to make sure that the abortion is completed
- Successful abortion cannot be confirmed immediately
- MTX is not approved by the FDA for this purpose but can still be given by your clinician

WHAT ARE THE RISKS OF MEDICAL ABORTION WITH MTX?

- Ongoing pregnancy
- Incomplete abortion
- Hemorrhage (severe bleeding) requiring a surgical procedure on the uterus
- Infection

WHO CAN USE MEDICAL ABORTION WITH MTX?

Women who:

- Had their last period at least 49 days ago (7 weeks) and no more than 63 days ago (9 weeks), and want or need to end the pregnancy
- Have given informed consent
- Are willing to abstain from sexual intercourse and alcohol for the first 14 days after the procedure and who will go to all appointments
- Have normal blood test results and do not have anemia (low blood cell count)

WHAT SHOULD I DO BEFORE A MEDICAL ABORTION WITH MTX?

- Consider and discuss alternatives (your clinician will have referrals for adoption and prenatal care)
- You will need to find a clinic that will prescribe the medicines and provide ongoing follow-up
- You will need to sign an informed consent form
- You should receive emotional support, education, and pre- and post-abortion instructions from a health care provider

WHAT SHOULD I DO AFTER A MEDICAL ABORTION WITH MTX?

- Expect moderate (sometimes severe) cramping, bleeding and nausea
- Do not have sexual intercourse or drink alcohol for 14 days; do not take vitamins that contain folate during treatment
- Either return for misoprostol or take it at home according to the schedule your clinician gives you
- Use a pain reliever such as ibuprofen for pain
- Have a support person close by after misoprostol is given
- Call your clinician if you have heavy bleeding (soaking 4 sanitary pads within 2 hours)
- Take medicine to prevent nausea, vomiting and diarrhea
- Use contraception in future sexual activity if you do not want to get pregnant

WHAT HAPPENS IF:

I have pain? You can take pain relief medicines such as aspirin, Tylenol or ibuprofen. You can also request stronger medicine for severe pain (usually after your clinician has evaluated you). In one study, 1 out of 300 women needed an injection for pain relief *[Creinin, 1997]*.

I have bleeding? Contact your clinician if bleeding becomes severe (more than your normal period). Surgical abortion procedure may be necessary if you are bleeding more than your normal period.

I have nausea/vomiting/diarrhea? Treat with anti-nausea/vomiting medicine (e.g., Dramamine) and anti-diarrhea medicine (e.g., Lomotil).

WHAT IF I WANT TO GET PREGNANT AFTER A MEDICAL ABORTION?
• Normal return to fertility
• No evidence of harm in future pregnancies due to these medicines

PREGNANCY TERMINATION:
MEDICAL ABORTION WITH MIFEPRISTONE (RU-486)

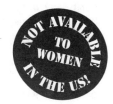

WHAT IS RU-486?
This kind of medical abortion uses a drug called RU-486, an abortion drug first used in France in 1989. When taken, it ends a pregnancy. RU-486 is not currently available in the U.S.

HOW EFFECTIVE IS RU-486?
• Mifepristone alone is about 80% effective
• Mifepristone followed by prostaglandin, a hormone that causes contractions, is about 95% effective within 48 hours if used in the 49 days since your last period began

HOW DOES RU-486 WORK?
RU-486 stops the hormone progesterone from continuing pregnancy.

HOW MUCH DOES RU-486 COST?
Will probably cost the same as a first-trimester surgical abortion.

WHAT ARE THE ADVANTAGES OF RU-486?
• Avoids risks of being given anesthesia during surgical abortion
• Reduces risk of cervical or uterine injury because there are no instruments in uterus
• Abortions may be performed very early
• Greater privacy and control for patients
• Some patients feel medical abortion is more "natural"
• Probably less risk of infection

WHAT ARE THE DISADVANTAGES OF RU-486?
• Takes longer than surgical abortion (about the same as methotrexate)
• Long-term follow-up studies are not available
• Cramping, pain, sometimes nausea, vomiting, or diarrhea
• Little is known about the effect it has on the fetus if the abortion is unsuccessful
• May not treat ectopic pregnancy (as opposed to methotrexate)

WHAT ARE THE RISKS OF RU-486? *[Silvestre, 1990]*

- Incomplete abortion (2%)
- Ongoing pregnancy (1%)
- Hemorrhage requiring emergency surgery (less than 1%)
- Complications requiring blood transfusion (0.1%)
- Infection (0.1%)

WHO CAN USE RU-486?

Women who:
- *Began* their last period 49 days (or before) for all procedures
- *Began* last period up to 63 days ago for some procedures
- Are not severely anemic (low red blood cell count)
- Are not regular users of injected or oral corticosteroids
  (NOTE: Ask your clinician if you are unsure about any of these issues)

WHAT SHOULD I DO BEFORE I USE RU-486?

- Discuss all pregnancy options with a health care provider
- Confirm the date of your last period
- Discuss the advantages and disadvantages of surgical and medical abortion with your clinician (see the chart on following page for a comparison)
- Consider with your clinician a surgical backup if abortion with RU-486 is incomplete

WHAT SHOULD I DO AFTER I USE RU-486?

- Have a support person ready to help you
- Have ready access to a bathroom
- Expect cramping and bleeding; may take a pain reliever to help relieve pain
- Expect nausea, vomiting or diarrhea

WHAT HAPPENS IF:

I have cramping, pain or bleeding? Take a pain reliever (possibly a prescription drug with codeine if pain is severe).

If abortion is incomplete? You may need a second dose of misoprostol or possibly surgery.

WHAT IF I WANT TO GET PREGNANT AFTER USING RU-486?

Normal return to fertility after using RU-486.

**If you have any questions,
ask us at…
www.managingcontraception.com**

Comparison of Medical and Surgical Abortion

Many people are not aware of the differences between medical abortion and surgical abortion. This table will help you compare the advantages and disadvantages of these two methods. See text in this chapter for details.

ABORTION METHOD	ADVANTAGES	DISADVANTAGES
Medical Abortion: Methotrexate OR Mifepristone with Misoprostol	No instruments in uterus; no risk of cervical or uterine injury	Can be used for pregnancies up to 7-9 weeks only (at least 49 days and no more than 63 days since last period)
	No anesthesia needed; no anesthetic risks	Pain and bleeding like miscarriage or heavy period for up to 14 days. May lead to anemia (which is usually easily treated)
	May perform abortions very early	About 1% continue pregnancy and need surgical abortion procedure
	More private process	About 4% have an incomplete abortion and need surgical abortion procedure
	Not dependent on surgical skills of clinician	Long-term follow-up studies not available
	Probably less risk of infection	Nausea, vomiting, diarrhea, cramping
		Need access to a bathroom for up to 1-2 weeks
		Methotrexate can cause birth defects if abortion is incomplete (unknown if Misoprostol or RU-486 can have this effect); must confirm pregnancy has been terminated
Surgical Abortion: Suction curettage	Procedure may be completed in 1 session. Some settings require a visit before, a visit to perform the procedure, and a follow-up visit	Needs local or general anesthesia
	Can return to normal activities the next day. Delay sexual intercourse until follow-up visit	Women may fear surgery
	Risk of incomplete abortion is less than 1%	Cervical or uterine injury possible
	Continuation of pregnancy is rare	Skilled clinicians may not be available

"Take a break from the pill" is just one example of contraceptive advice that is usually unnecessary and unwise. There is a lot of advice about the timing of contraceptive methods—when to start, when to stop—that is too strict and may get in the way of people using methods consistently and correctly. The table on the next page presents some traditional advice about the timing of certain methods, the reasons for it, and the problems that can happen if this advice is followed. It also provides what we consider to be better advice to help you and your health care provider avoid being too rigid on contraceptive timing.

REMEMBER: Birth control pills can be used for emergency contraception. When it comes to timing emergency contraception, the sooner you start the method from the time you had unprotected intercourse, the more effective it is. Each 12 hour delay in starting emergency contraceptive pill treatment following unprotected sex decreases contraceptive effectiveness. Each woman exposed to the risk of an unintended pregnancy should have the actual pills she would use in an emergency AVAILABLE for immediate use and should UNDERSTAND how to use them in advance (see chapter 24 for more information on emergency contraception).

See Timing Advice Table on the following page.

The right time to start or resume contraception is when failure to do so has any chance of leading to consequences which may negatively impact your life. If you are sexually active and want to avoid unintended pregnancies, this means NOW!

METHOD	TRADITIONAL TIMING ADVICE	BASIS FOR ADVICE	PROBLEMS WITH ADVICE	BEST OR BETTER ADVICE
Oral Contra- ceptive Pills	Start pills the Sunday after your next period begins	Convenience: • All patients doing same thing • No periods on weekends • Period is a good sign of not being pregnant	• Pills are more effective if you begin on *first* day of your period • Pills can begin anytime in cycle if not pregnant	Start first day of next period or start today (if not pregnant). It is always best to start any contraceptive the day you see your clinician so that you can have immediate pregnancy protection
	After several years of pill use, take a break	Several years ago, clinicians felt that they did not know enough about long-term pill use/effects	• Pregnancy from stopping pills • Irregular periods or may not get periods • Lose noncontraceptive benefits	No limit on how long you can take pills. Tell your clinician if you have any changes or problems
	Wait 3 months after stopping pills to get pregnant	Increased accuracy of dating pregnancy	• Ultrasound may be used for dating • A single menstrual period is sufficient	Begin attempting conception after first normal period
Depo- Provera	If breastfeeding, wait until 6 weeks after birth for first Depo-Provera shot	Possible concerns: • Effect on baby • Effect on quality/quantity of milk	• Delay may cause confusion • Failure to get first shot may lead to unintended pregnancy	It is possible to start Depo-Provera when you leave the hospital and plan to breastfeed **IF** milk flow is established
	Depo-Provera must begin during a woman's period	Periods mean that a woman is not pregnant	• Too restrictive • Vaginal bleeding does not definitely exclude pregnancy	You can start Depo-Provera anytime in your cycle if you and your clinician are sure you are not pregnant. Use a backup method for 7 days if you are not having your period
IUD	Clinician must insert IUD during menstruation	Periods mean that a woman is not pregnant	• Too restrictive • Vaginal bleeding does not definitely mean you are not pregnant • The IUD is more likely to be expelled if it is put in during a woman's period • Women who have IUDs inserted in the middle of their cycles are less likely to get them taken out [*White, 1980*]	IUD can be inserted if your clinician is sure you are not pregnant. It is always best to start any chosen contraceptive the day you see a clinician
	Remove Copper T 380-A after 4, 6, 8 or 10 years	Follows FDA labeling if removed after 10 years	Since first approved, labeling has called for removal at 4,6,8, then 10 years. Appears to be effective for longer than 10 years	Current advice should be: "Your IUD is effective for at least 10 years and may be effective longer"
Male Condom	Put condom on the erect penis	• Easier to put on • Erection happens before intercourse	• Couples might never put condom on once penis is erect • Foreplay may increase risk of infection	Put on condom anytime before insertion of penis in vagina, anus, or mouth. Partner can stimulate penis to erection with condom on

- Usually you will be able to use the method <u>YOU</u> want—tell your clinician what you want
- Each contraceptive method has both advantages and disadvantages
- Effectiveness and safety are important concerns (see page 36)
- Protection against STIs/HIV needs to be considered
- Convenience and ability to use method correctly are important
- Negotiation with your partner may be important
- Effects of method on your or your partner's period may be very important
- The best method is usually the one you will use consistently and correctly
- Other influences (religion, privacy, past experiences) may affect your choice

Effectiveness/failure data are presented in 2 ways (see page 35):

Perfect-use failure rate in first year: Among users who start using a method (not necessarily for the first time) and who use it perfectly (both consistently and correctly), the percentage who experience an accidental pregnancy during the first year.

Typical-use failure rate in first year: Among typical users who start using a method (not necessarily for the first time), the percentage who experience an accidental pregnancy during the first year. A population of typical users includes people who used the method perfectly and people who used the method incorrectly and inconsistently (e.g., forgetting to take pills, not using condoms everytime).

A key question to ask yourself and your partner: What would you do if you had an unintended pregnancy? Your answer to this question—be it abortion, keeping the baby, adoption—can help guide your method choice. For example, if you are absolutely sure you do not want an abortion if you get pregnant, you probably want to use a method that is close to 100% effective. It is also helpful to keep some statistics in mind, such as: **1)** the likelihood that you will get pregnant for each act of sexual intercourse, **2)** the risk of gonorrhea or chlamydia infection per act of intercourse, **3)** the likelihood that one of these infections will lead to PID (see below), and **4)**the risk of infertility after one or more episodes of pelvic inflammatory disease (PID)

A Look at the Risks from Unprotected Sex and Infections

1)Risk of pregnancy per act of intercourse	3)Risk of PID per woman infected with gonorrhea
17%-30% if woman is midcycle Less than 1% if during a woman's period	40% if not treated NO risk if PID is promptly & adequately treated

2)Risk of gonorrhea infection per act of intercourse	4)Risk of tubal infertility per PID episode
50% if infected male, uninfected female 25% if infected female, uninfected male	8% after first PID episode 20% after second PID episode 40% after third or greater PID episode

Cates W Jr. Reproductive tract infections. In: Hatcher RA, et al. Contraceptive Technology. 17th ed. New York: Ardent Media, 1998:181.

Percentage of U.S. women experiencing an unintended pregnancy within the first year of typical use or the first year of perfect use and the percentage continuing use at the end of the first year*:

Method	% of Women Experiencing an Unintended Pregnancy within the First Year of Use		% of Women or couples still using this method one year after starting[3]
	Typical Use[1]	Perfect Use[2]	
Chance (no contraceptive)	85	85	
Spermicides	26	6	40
Periodic Abstinence	25		63
Calendar		9	
Ovulation Method		3	
Symptothermal		2	
Post-ovulation		1	
Prentif Cap with spermicide			
Women who have given birth	40	26	42
Women who have NOT given birth	20	9	56
Sponge			
Women who have given birth	40	20	42
Women who have NOT given birth	20	9	56
Diaphragm with spermicide	20	6	56
Withdrawal	19	4	
Condom without spermicide			
Female (Reality)	21	5	56
Male (Latex)	14	3	61
Pill			
Progestin-only	5	0.5	
Combined	5	0.1	
IUD			
Progesterone T	2.0	1.5	81
Copper T 380A	0.8	0.6	78
Levonorgestrel	0.1	0.1	81
Depo-Provera (injection)	0.3	0.3	42
Norplant and Norplant-2	0.05	0.05	88
Female Sterilization	0.5	0.5	100
Male Sterilization	0.15	0.10	100

Emergency Contraceptive Pills: Treatment started within 72 hours after unprotected intercourse reduces the risk of pregnancy by at least 75%.

[1]Among typical couples who start using a method (not necessarily for the first time), the percentage who experience an accidental pregnancy during the first year if they do not stop use for any other reason.

[2]Among couples who start using a method (not necessarily for the first time) and who use it perfectly (both consistently and correctly), the percentage who experience an accidental pregnancy during the first year if they do not stop use for any other reason.

NOTE: For other footnotes to this table, see *Contraceptive Technology, A Pocket Guide to Managing Contraception*, or the package insert of most oral contraceptive pill.

*Trussell J, Kowal D. The essentials of contraception. In: Hatcher RA, et al. *Contraceptive Technology*, 17th ed. New York: Ardent Media, 1998:216-7. Slight adaptations from CT table.

Major methods of contraception and some related safety concerns, side effects, and noncontraceptive benefits

METHOD	DANGERS	SIDE EFFECTS	NONCONTRACEPTIVE BENEFITS *
Pill	Cardiovascular complications (stroke, heart attack, blood clots, high blood pressure), depression, liver tumors, possible increased risk of breast and cervical cancers	Nausea, headaches, dizziness, spotting, weight gain, breast tenderness, chloasma ("mask of pregnancy")	Decreases menstrual pain, PMS, and blood loss; protects against symptomatic PID, some cancers (ovarian, endometrial), some benign tumors (fibroids, benign breast masses), ectopic pregnancies and ovarian cysts; reduces acne
IUD	PID following insertion, uterine perforation, anemia	Menstrual cramping, increased bleeding spotting	Copper-T and LNg IUDs prevent ectopic pregnancies; progestin-releasing IUDs decrease menstrual blood loss and pain
Male Condom	Anaphylactic reaction to latex (severe allergic reaction)	Decreased sensation, genital irritation from allergy to latex, loss of spontaneity, noisy	Helps protect against STIs, including HIV; may delay premature ejaculation
Female Condom	None known	Uncomfortable for some users	Helps protect against STIs
Implant	Infection at implant site, complicated removals, depression	Tenderness at site, menstrual changes, hair loss, weight gain, headaches	Lactation not disturbed, may decrease menstrual cramps, pain, and blood loss
Injectable (progestin-only)	Depression, allergic reactions, excessive weight gain, possible bone loss	Menstrual changes, weight gain, headaches, adverse effects on cholesterol levels	Lactation not disturbed, reduces risk of seizures, may have protective effects against PID and ovarian and endometrial cancers
Sterilization	Infection, anesthetic complications, internal bleeding if pregnancy occurs after tubal sterilization, high risk that it will be ectopic	Pain at surgical site, psychological reactions, subsequent regret that the procedure was performed	Tubal sterilization reduces risk of ovarian cancer and may protect against PID
Abstinence	None known	Negotiation with partner may be difficult	Prevents infections, including HIV
Barriers: Diaphragm,	Vaginal and urinary tract infections, toxic shock syndrome	Pelvic pressure, vaginal irritation, vaginal discharges if left in too long, allergy	Provides modest protection against STIs
Cap, Sponge, Spermicides	Vaginal and urinary tract infections	Vaginal irritation, allergy	Provides modest protection against STIs
Lactational Amenorrhea Method (LAM)	Risk of HIV transmission to infant if mother HIV+	5% of women who breastfeed develop mastitis (infection of the breast)	Provides excellent nutrition for infants and is recommended by the American Academy of Pediatrics. Helps mother's uterus return to non-pregnant state

*Trussell J, Kowal D. The essentials of contraception. In Hatcher RA, et al. *Contraceptive Technology*. 17th ed. New York: Ardent Media, 1998:235. Slight adaptations from original table.

10 Tips on Staying Committed to Abstinence

1 Discuss your decision to abstain openly with your partner in the beginning of the relationship.

2 Discuss which activities you will abstain from and why.

3 Identify alternative activities to express intimacy.

4 Know that you can remain abstinent and be erotic and sexual (for ideas, see the list of 99 sexual things you can do while staying infection-free just before the Sexually Transmitted Infections chapter)

5 Identify possible "roadblocks" to abstinence and strategies to overcome them.

6 Work together to set sexual limits and communicate them during sexual activity.

7 Continue to discuss your commitment to abstinence with your partner throughout your relationship.

8 Get informed about and have methods of contraception and infection protection on hand in case the time comes when you decide not to abstain.

9 Know that emergency contraception is available if you were not able to or decided not to abstain.

10 Be proud of your commitment—whether it's based on values or a desire to prevent unintended pregnancy or infection.

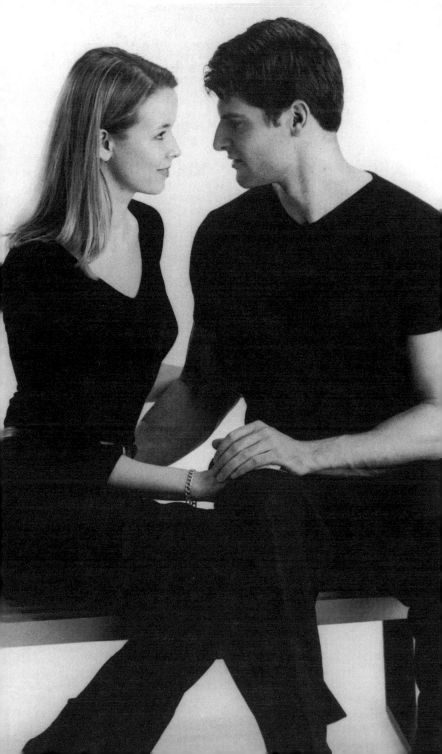

Abstinence

JUST SAY NO...TO WHAT?

There are many answers to the question "What is abstinence?" In family planning, abstinence from the activity that causes pregnancy is abstinence from penis-in-vagina intercourse. When it comes to protecting yourself from infection, abstinence means not exchanging body fluids (semen, vaginal fluids, blood, and breast milk) with another person. This includes abstaining from vaginal, anal, and oral intercourse, and any other activity (such as mutual masturbation) that might bring body fluids or infected areas of skin into contact. See previous pages for tips on staying committed to abstinence.

HOW EFFECTIVE IS ABSTINENCE?

Perfect-use failure rate in first year: 0%
Typical-use failure rate in first year: This has not been studied

HOW DOES ABSTINENCE WORK?

• No introduction of the penis or semen into the vagina prevents sperm from joining egg

HOW MUCH DOES ABSTINENCE COST? Nothing, it's free

WHAT ARE THE ADVANTAGES OF ABSTINENCE?

Menstrual:
• None, because there are no hormonal side effects
Sexual/psychological:
• May increase self-esteem and positive self-image if you feel that it is the best practice for you at a certain point in your life
• May increase creativity in ways to express intimacy
Cancers, tumors, and masses:
• Less risk of cervical cancer from HPV infection
Other:
• Protection against infections (best protection if no vaginal, anal, or oral intercourse)
• No medical side effects
• Many religions approve of abstinence at various times in people's lives
• Can be started at any time
• Nothing to buy

WHAT ARE THE DISADVANTAGES OF ABSTINENCE?

Menstrual: None
Sexual/psychological: Self-doubt; may feel as though you are "missing out"
Cancers, tumors, and masses: No impact

Other:
- •If only abstaining from penis-in-vagina intercourse, there may be no protection against infections transmitted through other activities such as oral and anal intercourse, including herpes, genital warts, gonorrhea, and HIV/AIDS
- •Requires commitment and self-control from both partners
- •Couples may not be prepared to protect themselves from pregnancy and STIs when they stop abstaining
- •Couples who change their minds may have little knowledge about contraception
- •One partner may pressure the other to have sex

WHAT ARE THE RISKS OF ABSTINENCE?
- No medical risks
- You may be in situations where you would like to abstain, but your partner does not agree. Individuals have been raped and beaten for refusing to have sex. Clearly this is wrong, but it can sometimes happen when one person wants to abstain and the other person refuses to accept that decision

WHO CAN USE ABSTINENCE?
- Individuals or couples who feel that they can control a sexual situation

What About Adolescents? Abstinence is an excellent method for adolescents. They need skills and information on how to handle peer pressure and need to know about contraceptives and possibly have a method available in case abstinence is not chosen or not possible. Individuals counting on abstinence as their contraceptive need to know about emergency contraception should a mistake happen or should an adolescent be forced to have intercourse.

HOW DO I START OR RETURN TO USING ABSTINENCE?
- Individuals need to commit to abstaining and discuss it beforehand with sexual partners. Do not simply assume abstinence. It is a lot more than "just saying no"
- It is possible to "return to abstinence" after being sexually active or after giving birth

WHAT GUIDELINES SHOULD I FOLLOW?
- Establish ground rules in advance for yourself and your partner
- Discuss with your partner and make a plan for if and when the time comes when you will be sexually active
- Drugs and alcohol can greatly affect the choice to abstain. Being drunk or using other drugs may make either partner less likely to stick with abstinence
- Have condoms and emergency contraception on hand in case of emergency

WHAT HAPPENS IF:
My partner does not want to abstain? You will need to negotiate openly with him or her. Talking to a health care provider (alone or together with your partner) may be helpful. ***It is also very important to have a back-up contraceptive plan.***

WHAT IF I WANT TO GET PREGNANT AFTER ABSTAINING?
Abstinence protects your future fertility because it can greatly reduce your risk of getting an infection that can lead to infertility.

HOW CAN BREASTFEEDING BE A CONTRACEPTIVE METHOD?

Breastfeeding can be a temporary method of contraception when the baby's diet is 90%-100% breast milk, when periods have not returned (spotting that occurs in the first 56 days after birth is not regarded as regular periods), and when the newborn is less than 6 months old. Women who breastfeed less completely, whose periods have returned, and whose babies are more than 6 months old, need to add additional methods to protect against pregnancy.

HOW EFFECTIVE IS EXCLUSIVE, FULL BREASTFEEDING AS CONTRACEPTION?

Perfect-use failure rate in first 6 months of baby's life: 0.5%
Typical-use failure rate in first 6 months of baby's life: 2% *[Kennedy, 1998]*
At any time, emergency contraception (COCs or POPs) may be used by a nursing mother if she or clinician is concerned that she is at risk for pregnancy.

HOW DOES BREASTFEEDING WORK AS CONTRACEPTION?

A baby sucking on the mother's nipple causes a surge in the hormone prolactin in the mother's blood. Prolactin hormone stops ovulation.

HOW MUCH DOES BREASTFEEDING COST? Nothing, it's free

WHAT ARE THE ADVANTAGES OF BREASTFEEDING AS CONTRACEPTION?

Menstrual:
- The uterus returns to normal more rapidly
- Monthly periods are suppressed

Sexual/psychological:
- Breastfeeding generally does not interfere with sex and breastfeeding may be pleasurable (physically and emotionally) for some women
- May help the mother and child bond

Cancers, tumors, and masses: Slight protective effect against ovarian and pre-menopausal breast cancer in the mother

Other:
- Can be used immediately after childbirth
- Provides the healthiest food for baby
- Helps protect baby against asthma, diarrhea, and ear infections because mother's immunities are passed through breast milk and the child is not exposed to bottle feeding until later in infancy
- May help the mother lose weight after birth

WHAT ARE THE DISADVANTAGES OF BREASTFEEDING AS CONTRACEPTION?

Menstrual: When fertility has returned is not always clear to a nursing woman (see page 42)
Sexual/psychological: May be initially embarrassing for some women to breastfeed
Cancers, tumors, and masses: None
Other:
- Effectiveness after 6 months is greatly reduced. Breastfeeding is not recommended as a contraceptive method after 6 months and another method should be used. Breastfeeding for baby's nutrition can, of course, continue indefinitely
- Frequent breastfeeding may be inconvenient for women

39

- If the mother is HIV-positive, there is a 14%-29% chance that HIV will be passed to her baby. Breastfeeding is not recommended for HIV-positive mothers who have other safe and healthy food available for their babies
- Some women may have an inadequate milk supply
- Sore nipples and breasts; risk of mastitis (breast infection)
- No protection against infections or HIV/AIDS; you must use condoms for protection

WHAT ARE THE RISKS OF BREASTFEEDING?
- 5% of women who breastfeed will develop mastitis (a breast infection)
- Nipple tenderness

IS BREASTFEEDING THE RIGHT CONTRACEPTIVE METHOD FOR ME?
If you answer "no" to all of the questions, breastfeeding is an effective form of contraception for you.

1. Is your baby 6 months old or older?

☐ No   ☐ Yes   You should not use breastfeeding alone as a contraceptive. You need to choose another method as a back-up.

2. Have your menstrual periods returned? (Bleeding in the first 8 weeks after childbirth does not count.)

☐ No   ☐ Yes   After 8 weeks after birth, if you have 2 straight days of menstrual-type bleeding, or your menstrual period has returned, breastfeeding as a contraceptive will be less effective. You need to choose another method.

3. Have you begun to breastfeed less often? Do you regularly give the baby other food or liquid?

☐ No   ☐ Yes   If the baby's feeding pattern has just changed, you must fully or nearly fully breastfeed to protect against pregnancy. Breastfeed often, day and night, and for almost all of your baby's feedings (90% or more is what is meant by fully breastfeeding). If you are not fully or nearly fully breastfeeding, it will not be as effective as a contraceptive. You need to choose another method.

4. Has a health care provider told you not to breastfeed your baby?

☐ No   ☐ Yes   You should not breastfeed if you are taking certain mood-altering drugs (reserpine, ergotamine, antimetabolites, cyclosporine, cortisone, bromocriptine, radioactive drugs, lithium, or certain anticoagulants) or if you are HIV-positive or carry viral hepatitis. All others can and should consider breastfeeding for the health benefits for you and your baby. Ask your health care provider if you are not sure.

5. Do you have AIDS? Are you infected with HIV, the virus that causes AIDS?

☐ No   ☐ Yes   In the United States, where safe alternatives to feeding a baby are available, breastfeeding your infant is discouraged if you are HIV-positive as breastmilk may transmit HIV to your baby. In countries where infectious diseases kill many babies, it may be wise even for mothers who are infected with HIV to breastfeed because breast milk helps increase the baby's immune system.

WHO CAN USE BREASTFEEDING AS A CONTRACEPTIVE?
- Women who are fully breastfeeding (at least 90% of nutrition comes from breast milk)
- Women with children less than 6 months old
- Women who have not had a return of periods

What About Adolescents? This method can be used by adolescents who are committed to breastfeeding without giving their babies other food for the first 6 months.

WHAT GUIDELINES SHOULD I FOLLOW?
- Breastfeed consistently without giving your baby other food for maximum effectiveness
- Breast milk should make up at least 90% of baby's feedings

HOW DO I START THE METHOD?
- Start breastfeeding immediately after birth and make sure you are breastfeeding fully or almost fully (at least 90% of baby's feedings should be breast milk)
- *If you definitely do not want to become pregnant, it is a good idea to use a second method of contraception as a back-up*

WHAT HAPPENS IF:
I do not make enough milk?
- Immediately after birth you should breastfeed every 1 -2 hours
- Breastfeed often (8-10 times a day), get additional rest, take in lots of fluids and iron-rich foods and/or supplements
- This is commonly caused by not enough nursing, use of an artificial nipple, fatigue or stress

I have sore nipples?
- Commonly caused by incorrect positioning of the baby to the breast
- Inquire about correct ways of latching and sucking
- Improves with practice
- Cleanse nipples before and after sucking to reduce infection and nipple soreness
- Application of breast milk to nipple after cleansing may help

I have sore breasts?
- Apply heat on sore areas
- Nurse frequently or use pump to get excess milk out of sore breast
- Get more rest
- You need to speak with or be examined by your clinician if you also have a fever, a particular area of redness, or a very localized area of severe tenderness

Other:
- Stress, fear, lack of confidence, lack of family or societal support, and/or poor nutrition can cause problems (ask your clinician if you are unsure or have any problems)

WHAT IF I WANT TO GET PREGNANT AFTER USING BREASTFEEDING AS CONTRACEPTION?
Breastfeeding has no effect on future fertility and the return of fertility is normal. If your clinician agrees, you can continue to breastfeed while you are pregnant. However, milk supply often diminishes after conception.

CAN I USE BREASTFEEDING AS A CONTRACEPTIVE?

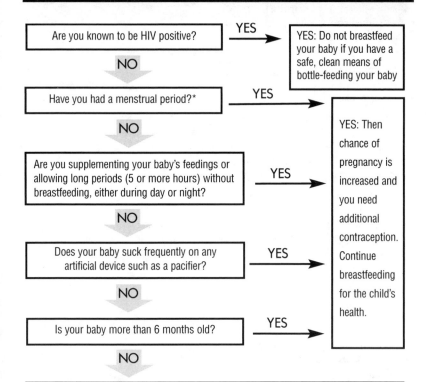

Are you known to be HIV positive?

NO

YES → YES: Do not breastfeed your baby if you have a safe, clean means of bottle-feeding your baby

Have you had a menstrual period?*

NO

YES →

Are you supplementing your baby's feedings or allowing long periods (5 or more hours) without breastfeeding, either during day or night?

NO

YES →

Does your baby suck frequently on any artificial device such as a pacifier?

NO

YES →

Is your baby more than 6 months old?

NO

YES →

YES: Then chance of pregnancy is increased and you need additional contraception. Continue breastfeeding for the child's health.

Then breastfeeding will be an effective contraceptive (only a 1% to 2% chance of pregnancy) until your baby is 6 months old.

*Spotting that occurs in the first 56 days after birth is <u>not</u> a menstrual period.

Source: Adapted significantly from Labbok M, et al, 1994. Institute of Reproductive Health, Georgetown University. Washington DC. Breastfeeding definitely can lead to transmission of HIV from mother to infant. If a safe, clean alternative to breast milk is available breastfeeding should be avoided. A question about HIV status is not included in the Labbok/Institute of Reproductive Health algorithm. Nor is the question about extensive use of a pacifier.

NOTE: In the United States the customary length of breastfeeding is about 3 months. Breastfeeding women do not know when their periods will return, when they will start giving other foods to their babies or exactly when they will stop breastfeeding their infant. Nor do they know if the first ovulation will precede or follow the first menstrual bleeding. It is wise to have a contraceptive you will use when the answer to one of the above questions becomes "yes" and to have a backup contraceptive even during the period when breastfeeding is effective.

All breastfeeding women who have just given birth should be provided contraception options because:

- It is still possible for ovulation to occur in breastfeeding women who have not resumed monthly periods
- Length of breastfeeding in the United States is quite brief in many women
- Most U.S. couples start having intercourse soon after birth

When to initiate contraception in breastfeeding women: Talk these options over with your partner and your clinician

METHOD	WHEN TO START IN BREASTFEEDING WOMEN	EFFECT ON BREAST MILK
Barrier Methods	• Immediately if maximum protection against pregnancy is desired *	• No effect
Combined Pills	• As a mother begins to wean her baby from breast milk; some disagreement among experts • When a mother begins to give her baby other food; some disagreement among experts • When a woman is fully or almost fully breastfeeding; a lot of disagreement among experts	• Changes can occur in quantity and composition of breast milk
Progestin-Only Methods • Depo-Provera • Progestin-Only Pills • Norplant	• Planned Parenthood Federation of America considers it appropriate for women to initiate any progestin-only methods immediately postpartum • World Health Organization and International Planned Parenthood Federation recommend waiting until 6 weeks after birth to initiate progestin-only methods if a woman is breastfeeding	• Progestins may increase milk flow
IUD	• May insert IUD immediately after birth until 48 hrs after birth • Avoid insertion from 48 hrs to 4 wks after birth • May carefully insert IUD from 4 wks after birth and later	• No effect
Tubal Sterilization	• Anytime after birth; may be most easily done 1-2 days after birth. (often this is covered for non-insured patients during this time)	• No effect

* Except for diaphragms and cervical caps which must be fit after the cervix returns to normal. Condoms and spermicides may be used as soon as it is safe to have intercourse. Sponges may be used after uterine bleeding stops.

WHAT IS NATURAL FAMILY PLANNING (NFP) OR THE RHYTHM METHOD?

Natural family planning methods use physical signs, symptoms, and menstrual cycle data to determine when ovulation occurs. During the time of the month when the woman is likely to get pregnant, the couple abstains from sexual intercourse or uses barrier methods. Natural family planning requires commitment and careful attention to monitoring the woman's cycle changes. It is most effective with excellent support and education. You will find resources to help you use this method at the end of this chapter. Because of the higher typical-use failure rates for those methods, tehy may not be appropriate for women with conditions which make pregnancy an unacceptable risk. Techniques used to determine high-risk pregnancy days include:

1. Calendar Method
- Before starting this method, record your periods for 6 cycles (6 months)
- Assume sperm can survive 3 days and ovulation occurs 14 days before first day of bleeding during period
- Earliest day of fertile period = number days of shortest cycle length minus 18
- Latest day of fertile period = number days of longest cycle length minus 11
- The following table will help you calculate your fertile days. You may also want to go to one of the websites explaining the natural family planning methods in more detail (see pages ix-x)

Charting Menstrual Cycles: How to Calculate Fertile Days

If your shortest cycle has been	Your first fertile day is:	If your longest cycle has been:	Your last fertile day is:
21	3rd day	21	10th day
22	4th	22	11th
23	5th	23	12th
24	6th	24	13th
25	7th	25	14th
26	8th	26	15th
27	9th	27	16th
28	10th	28	17th
29	11th	29	18th
30	12th	30	19th
31	13th	31	20th
32	14th	32	21st
33	15th	33	22nd
34	16th	34	23rd
35	17th	35	24th

Day 1 = First day of menstrual bleeding   Stewart F., Guest F. et al. *Understanding Your Body.* Bantam Books, 1987, p. 89.

2. Cervical Mucus Ovulation Detection Method
- Woman checks quantity and character of mucus on the vulva or vaginal opening with fingers or tissue paper each day for several months to learn cycle.
  Here are the types of mucus:
  - Post-menstrual fertile mucus: scant or undetectable
  - Pre-ovulation fertile mucus: cloudy, yellow or white, sticky
  - Ovulation mucus: thick, slippery, clear
  - Post-ovulation fertile mucus: thick, cloudy, sticky
  - Post-ovulation post-fertile mucus: scant or undetectable
- When using this method during the pre-ovulatory period, wait 24 hours after intercourse to make test accurate
- Use abstinence or a barrier method during the 4-day fertile period
- Intercourse without restriction only during post-ovulatory infertile periods
- NOTE: Douching, having a vaginal infection, and using vaginal spermicides will make it difficult to interpret cervical mucus

44

3. Basal Body Temperature Method (BBT)
- Uses a digital thermometer to monitor a woman's temperature. Assume that body temperature will increase noticeably (0.4-0.8 F) at ovulation. The fertile period is defined as the day of the first drop or first elevation through 3 consecutive days of elevated temperature
- Temperature may not be accurate if a woman is sick and has a fever

Basal body temperature changes during a menstrual cycle

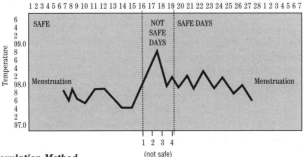

4. Post-ovulation Method
- Permits unprotected intercourse only after signs of ovulation have subsided. This is the most effective natural family planning method

5. Symptothermal Method
- Combines at least two methods — usually cervical mucus changes with BBT
- May also include mittelschmerz (sharp pain in the lower abdomen that some women get at ovulation), change in libido, and changes in cervical texture, position and dilation:
  - In pre-ovulatory and ovulatory periods, cervix is softer, more moist and slightly open
  - In post-ovulatory period, cervix drops, becomes firm and closes

HOW EFFECTIVE IS NATURAL FAMILY PLANNING?

| | First-year failure rate | |
Method	Typical use	Perfect use
Calendar	25%	9%
Ovulation Method	25	3
Symptothermal	25	2
Post-ovulation	25	1

[Trussell, Contraceptive Technology, 1998]

HOW DOES NATURAL FAMILY PLANNING WORK? Abstinence or barriers during fertile periods prevent sperm from entering vagina.

HOW MUCH DOES NATURAL FAMILY PLANNING COST? Training, supplies (digital thermometer), and barrier methods may cost money (amount depends on where supplies and training are obtained).

WHAT ARE THE ADVANTAGES OF NATURAL FAMILY PLANNING?
Menstrual:
- Helps woman learn more about her menstrual physiology
- No side effects or complications from hormones

Sexual/psychological: Men and women can work together in using this method
Cancers, tumors, and masses: None
Other:
- May be only method acceptable to couples for cultural or religious reasons
- Helps couples achieve pregnancy when practiced in reverse

45

WHAT ARE THE DISADVANTAGES OF NATURAL FAMILY PLANNING?

Menstrual:
- Works poorly for those with irregular or unpredictable menstrual cycles
- Difficult to use when approaching menopause and in women who have given birth and have irregular (or absent) cycles

Sexual/psychological:
- It takes at least 6 months of recording cycles to learn how to use natural family planning. During this time, you must abstain from sex or use a barrier method
- If you are using the basal body temperature method and no ovulation occurs, you must abstain from sex completely or use other methods carefully
- Requires discipline, good communication, and full commitment of both partners
- Requires abstinence or a barrier method at the time of ovulation, which is often the time of peak sexual desire

Cancers, tumors, and masses: None

Other:
- Does not protect against sexually transmitted infections
- Often unreliable during time of stress or illness because cycles may be irregular
- Risk of pregnancy is high if improper use
- Relatively high failure rate

WHAT ARE THE RISKS OF NATURAL FAMILY PLANNING?

None, except the relatively higher risk of pregnancy.

WHO CAN USE NATURAL FAMILY PLANNING?

- Highly motivated users willing to commit to periods of abstinence or to use barriers during high risk periods
- Those with religious/cultural proscription against using other methods

What About Adolescents? Not appropriate until periods are regular and until they have developed the discipline and communication that is necessary.

IS NATURAL FAMILY PLANNING THE RIGHT CONTRACEPTIVE METHOD FOR ME?

Ask yourself the questions below. If you answer NO to ALL questions, you CAN use any fertility awareness-based method you want. If you answer YES to any question, follow the instructions. No conditions restrict use of these methods, but some conditions can make them harder to use effectively.

1. Do you have a medical condition that would make pregnancy especially dangerous?

☐ No   ☐ Yes   If yes, you may want to choose a more effective method. If not, you must use fertility awareness-based methods carefully to avoid pregnancy.

2. Do you have irregular menstrual cycles? Vaginal bleeding between periods? Heavy or long monthly bleeding?
For younger women: Are your periods just starting?
For older women: Have your periods become irregular, or have they stopped?

☐ No   ☐ Yes   Predicting your fertile time with only the calendar method may be hard or impossible. You can use basal body temperature (BBT) and/or cervical mucus, or you may prefer another method.

3. Did you recently give birth or have an abortion? Are you breastfeeding? Do you have any other condition that affects the ovaries or menstrual bleeding, such as: stroke, serious liver disease, thyroid disease, or cervical cancer?

☐ No   ☐ Yes   These conditions do not restrict use of fertility awareness-based methods, but they may affect fertility signs, making fertility awareness-based methods hard to use. For this reason, you may prefer a different method. If not, you may need extra training to make sure you know how to use the method optimally.

4. Do you have any infections or diseases that may change cervical mucus, basal body temperatures, or menstrual bleeding—such as sexually transmitted infections (STI) or pelvic inflammatory disease (PID) in the last 3 months, or vaginal infections?

☐ No   ☐ Yes   These conditions may affect fertility signs, making natural family planning methods hard to use. Once an infection is treated and reinfection is avoided, however, you can use natural family planning methods more easily.

5. Do you take any drugs that affect your menstrual cycle or cervical mucus, such as mood-altering drugs, lithium, tricyclic anti-depressants, or anti-anxiety therapies?

☐ No   ☐ Yes   Predicting your fertile time correctly may be difficult or impossible if you use only the cervical mucus method or the calendar method. You may prefer another method.

6. Do you have irregular periods because you have recently stopped using Depo-Provera?

☐ No   ☐ Yes   If your cycles have not become regular yet, you should use another method until they do.

HOW DO I START NATURAL FAMILY PLANNING?
• Requires several months of data collection and analysis and practice before a couple can begin using this method as their primary method of contraception
• It is necessary for individuals interested in these methods to get formal counseling and education. Resources for these methods are listed below:
  California Family Health Council: 3600 Wilshire Boulevard, Suite 20 Los Angeles CA, 90010 Tel: 626-931-1400 or on the Internet at www.cfhc.org
  The Couple to Couple League Foundation: P.O. Box 11184 Cincinnati, Ohio 45211 Tel: 513-471-2000

WHAT GUIDELINES SHOULD I FOLLOW?
• Requires discipline, communication, listening skills, and full commitment of both partners
• Abstain from sex or use barrier contraception during fertile days
• Effectiveness of natural family planning can be greatly reduced by the use of drugs or alcohol

WHAT HAPPENS IF:
I have had intercourse during "unsafe" times in my cycle? You may want to use emergency contraception if you are concerned about being pregnant (see chapter 24, page 68).

WHAT IF I WANT TO GET PREGNANT AFTER USING NATURAL FAMILY PLANNING?
• Natural family planning has no effect on future fertility
• Some couples who want to get pregnant use fertility awareness techniques to maximize their chances

Condoms 101

You've probably heard a lot about responsibility, maturity, and discipline when it comes to using condoms. Well, there's something else you need to know... condoms can be fun, too!

Condoms come in different colors, shapes, sizes, and flavors—blue, green, yellow, glow in the dark, medium, extra sensitive, superduper extra large, ribbed, lubricated, nonlubricated, mint, orange, banana, pina colada, and grape. The possibilities are endless!

You might try a different type of condom each time you have sex, or you could use a flavored condom during oral sex. If you're concerned that putting on a condom will "ruin the moment," try putting one on as a part of foreplay. You may be pleasantly surprised...

Finally, remember that the experience of using condoms, as with all contraceptive methods, can be shared between men and women. It takes two committed partners to have safe—and pleasurable—sex!

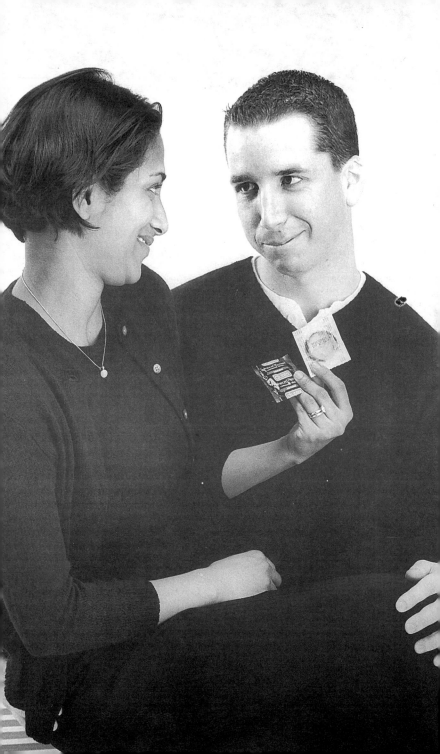

WHAT ARE MALE CONDOMS?

Condoms are sheaths made of latex, polyurethane (plastic), or natural membranes (from sheep intestine). Polyurethane condoms may be used by couples when either partner is allergic to latex. Used correctly, condoms are effective in preventing both pregnancy and infection. Check out www.condomania.com to see a colorful display of condom options.

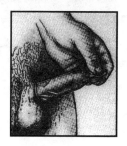

HOW EFFECTIVE ARE MALE LATEX CONDOMS?

Perfect-use failure rate in first year: 3%
Typical-use failure rate in first year: 14%
Continuing users after one year: 61%   *[Trussell J, Contraceptive Technology 1998]*

- Condoms usually "fail" because they are not used NOT because they break or slip
- Most studies report breakage rates less than 2%; less than 1 break in 100 acts of intercourse has been reported in experienced users
- Condoms have been shown in several studies to be several times more likely to slip down or fall off than they are to break
- Numerous studies show that condoms are highly effective in protecting against HIV and other infections. They are not perfect, but they work. (for more information, see www.jsi.com/intl/fpln/pdf/condomresponse.pdf)

HOW DO CONDOMS WORK?

Condoms act as a mechanical barrier; they prevent pregnancy by stopping sperm from going into the vagina.

Condoms and Spermicides: "Whether condoms lubricated with spermicides are more effective than other lubricated condoms in protecting against the transmission of HIV and other STDs has not been determined. Furthermore, spermicide-coated condoms have been associated with *Escherichia coli* urinary tract infection in women." *[Centers for Disease Control, 1998]*

HOW MUCH DO CONDOMS COST?

Costs range from free at many clinics and HIV programs to several dollars for a designer condom. Average retail cost of a latex condom is $.50 and for the polyurethane Avanti condom is $2. There is also a new polyurethane condom called Trojan Supra. A box of natural skin condoms costs about $20.

WHAT ARE THE ADVANTAGES OF CONDOMS?

Menstrual: Safe; no hormonal side effects
Sexual/psychological:
- Sexual intercourse may be enjoyed more because there is less fear of STIs, HIV, and pregnancy
- Men can be involved
- Men "last longer" when they use condoms, which might make sex more fun
- Come in many sizes, colors, shapes, flavors, and packaging; variety can be exciting
- If the man's partner puts the condom on it can be fun (for both partners)
- Risk of infertility for partner is decreased (because less risk of infection)
Cancers, tumors, and masses:
- May reduce risk of cervical cancer (because less risk of HPV infection)

Other:
- Makes sex less messy by catching the ejaculate
- No medical visit needed
- Fairly easy to get; usually do not cost a lot
- Good option during breastfeeding or with other methods as a backup

WHAT ARE THE DISADVANTAGES OF CONDOMS?

Menstrual: Offers none of the potential benefits of hormonal contraceptives
Sexual/psychological:
- Requires some practice to learn how to use
- Either partner must feel comfortable placing the condom on the penis
- Buying, negotiating use, putting on, and getting rid of condoms may be embarrassing for some people
- Unless put on by the partner as part of foreplay, it may interrupt sex
- Possible decreased enjoyment of sex from decreased sensation (for either partner)
- Some men cannot maintain an erection once the condom is on

Cancers, tumors, and masses: None
Other:
- Typical-user failure rate in one year is 14%
- Some people are allergic to latex; they may use polyurethane condom (Avanti or Trojan Supra)
- Oil-based lubricants and oil-based vaginal products will cause holes latex condoms (see list below)
- Must be careful not to tear condom when putting it on
- Condom may break or slip
- May not be available when needed
- Opening condom package in the excitement of the moment may be difficult

DO NOT USE THESE LUBRICANTS AND VAGINAL PRODUCTS WITH LATEX CONDOMS (most on this list are oil-based)*

Baby oil
Cold creams
Edible oils (olive, peanut, corn, sunflower)
Hand and body lotions
Massage oils
Mineral oil
Petroleum jelly (Vaseline)
Rubbing alcohol
Shortening
Suntan oil and lotions
Whipped cream

Vegetable oil and cooking oils
Vaginal yeast infection medicines in cream or suppository form:
- Clindamycin 2% vaginal cream
- Butoconazole cream
- Clotrimazole cream
- Clotrimazole vaginal tablet
- Miconazole vaginal suppository
- Terconazole ointment
- Terconazole cream or vaginal suppository

* *These lubricants/vaginal products **can** be used with polyurethane condoms.*

DO USE THESE LUBRICANTS WITH LATEX CONDOMS

(lubricants which are not oil-based)

Water and saliva	H-R Lubricating Jelly	AquaLube	Ramses Personal Spermicide
Glycerin	K-Y Jelly	Astroglide	Touch Personal Lubricant
Spermicide	Prepair	ForPlay	Cornhuskers Lotion
Aloe-9	Probe	Gynol II	Silicone Lubricant
Liquid Silk	Egg Whites (uncooked)	Wet	deLube

WHAT ARE THE RISKS OF MALE CONDOMS?
- Allergic reactions to latex (rare but may be serious for either man or woman)
- Infection caused by leaving condom in vagina for a long time (if it becomes lost or forgotten)

ARE MALE CONDOMS THE RIGHT METHOD FOR ME?

1. Are you or your partner allergic to latex?

☐ No   ☐ Yes   If yes, do not use latex condoms. You can use Avanti or Trojan Supra polyurethane male condoms, polyurethane Reality female condoms, or natural skin condoms with or without other condoms to protect you or your partner from latex.

2. Are you or your partner unable to maintain an erection while using condoms?

☐ No   ☐ Yes   If yes, you may want to consider another method as this greatly reduces the effectiveness and interferes with sexual activity.

WHO CAN USE CONDOMS?

• Individuals wanting protection against pregnancy and/or infection
• Individuals willing to use only a single method when infection is a concern
• Men who want to last longer during intercourse before orgasm
• Individuals having sex in first few weeks after birth when pelvic infection is an important concern
• Pregnant women who are at risk for infection of any kind
• Women and men with herpes or genital warts (with and without signs of infection)

What About Adolescents? Excellent option for adolescents who are trained and motivated. It is best for adolescents to use condoms along with another contraceptive method (such as pills, Depo-Provera, or Norplant).

HOW DO I START USING CONDOMS?

Users need to commit themselves in advance to using condoms every single time. You can carry them in your wallet or purse, but not for longer than 1 month *[Glasser, G, Hatcher RA., 1992]*. You also need to keep them away from heat (including body heat) and sunlight. Obtain emergency contraception from your clinician in **advance** in case you need it.

WHAT GUIDELINES SHOULD I FOLLOW? Getting it right, exactly right (see page 52)

The biggest help is practice. Many of the following steps can be practiced using the man's own penis or a cucumber:

1. Store in a dry, cool place away from sunlight; heat will cause the condom to weaken
2. Note the expiration date or manufacture date on each condom; if past expiration date, throw away and get a new one. Most condoms can be used up to 5 years after the *manufacture* date
3. Open package carefully to avoid tears
4. Avoid tearing condom with fingernails, rings, dental appliances, foil packaging or anything sharp
5. Avoid oil-based lubricants when using latex condoms
6. USE A WATER-BASED or SILICON-BASED LUBRICANT such as Astroglide, Wet or K-Y Jelly Plus Nonoxynol-9 (you can also use water or saliva) (see page 49); put this lubricant onto the surface of the condom and also inside the condom if desired; this helps to prevent condom breakage and may make sex more fun
7. Use two male condoms if worried about infection or pregnancy, particularly if either person might have an infection or has any discharge, sore, ulcer or signs of injection drug use such as needle marks; using two condoms is common among partners who have had a condom break in the past
8. If you use a latex male condom with a female condom, make sure to use extra water-based lubricant because the rubbing together can cause either condom to break or pull out. The oil-based lubricant in the female condom package may cause latex to break
9. The man's partner may put the condom on for him
10. Put condom on early in the course of sexual intimacy before genital contact; while pre-ejaculatory fluid ("pre-cum") usually has only nonmotile sperm, some men ejaculate with very little warning; pre-ejaculatory fluid may contain HIV and other STIs and penile skin can transmit HSV (Herpes) & HPV (virus that causes genital warts)
11. Refrain from rough or very vigorous sex; this can cause a condom to break

12. If you have oral or anal intercourse before vaginal intercourse, change condoms
13. Not all penises are the same. Penis size varies and so do condoms, so find a condom that is a comfortable fit for you (and your partner)
14. Some couples check the condition of the condom throughout sexual intercourse, especially if they have experienced a break in the past, or if intercourse is particularly rough or lasts long
15. If in doubt about slippage or breakage, put on new condom or put a second one on top of first
16. Both the penis and condom should be pulled out of the vagina immediately after ejaculation; either partner should hold the rim of the condom during withdrawal so the condom does not slip off
17. Dispose of condom. Do not reuse! Do not flush it down toilet-it will clog plumbing!
18. When a condom does break, fall off, or slip down, you may call "1-888-NOT 2 LATE" to find the telephone numbers of the 5 nearest providers who will provide you or your partner with emergency contraception
19. **REMEMBER:** Consistent and correct use of male condoms can be greatly reduced by the use of drugs and alcohol. Being drunk or high might make you more likely to make mistakes or not use a condom at all

DO I NEED TO CONSULT MY CLINICIAN? ASK YOURSELF:

Following are important questions to help you evaluate your use of condoms. If you answer "yes" to any question, talk to your provider to figure out the best solution for you.

☐ Have I or my partner experienced any rash or discomfort?
☐ Have I had intercourse without using a condom (even once)?
☐ During intercourse have I experienced condom breakage or slippage?
☐ Do I want to have emergency contraception available?

WHAT HAPPENS IF:

I have an allergic reaction? Try using an Avanti male condom (polyurethane); or use a Reality female condom (polyurethane); or use both a latex and a natural membrane condom: If the man is allergic to latex, the natural membrane condom goes onto the penis first, then the latex condom. If the man's partner is allergic to latex, the latex condom goes onto the penis first, and is covered by the natural membrane condom.

The condom breaks or slips? If repeated condom breakage or slippage occurs, consider using a different condom, a different way of using the condom, or use of other contraceptives. If a mistake happens and a condom breaks, falls off, slips down, or is not used, refer to the figure below and to chapter 22 on emergency contraception.

WHAT IF I WANT TO GET PREGNANT AFTER USING CONDOMS?

• Condoms can help prevent the infections that cause infertility
• There is no delay in return to fertility

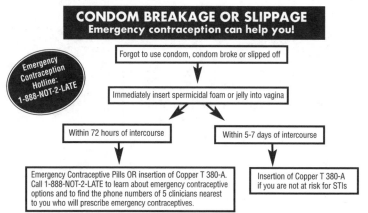

CONDOM BREAKAGE OR SLIPPAGE
Emergency contraception can help you!

Emergency Contraception Hotline: 1-888-NOT-2-LATE

Forgot to use condom, condom broke or slipped off

Immediately insert spermicidal foam or jelly into vagina

Within 72 hours of intercourse

Within 5-7 days of intercourse

Emergency Contraceptive Pills OR insertion of Copper T 380-A. Call 1-888-NOT-2-LATE to learn about emergency contraceptive options and to find the phone numbers of 5 clinicians nearest to you who will prescribe emergency contraceptives.

Insertion of Copper T 380-A if you are not at risk for STIs

"Many men hate condoms so much that they will pay a prostitute extra not to wear one. If they feel strongly about not wearing one with you, they probably have been exactly the same way with someone else—perhaps recently."

What I've Learned About Sex by Debra Haffner and Pepper Schwartz

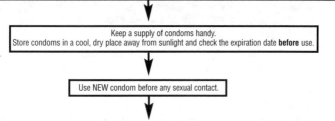

HOW TO USE A LATEX CONDOM
(...Or rubber, sheath, prophylactic, safe, french letter, raincoat, glove, sock)

Think and talk about condom use with partner. Make the FIRM commitment, in advance, to use condoms without exception at each and every act of vaginal intercourse (and including oral and anal intercourse when at risk of infection).

Keep a supply of condoms handy.
Store condoms in a cool, dry place away from sunlight and check the expiration date **before** use.

Use NEW condom before any sexual contact.

USE CONDOM CORRECTLY.
Before putting on the condom, check to see which way the condom unrolls.
Squeeze out all air in the 1/2-inch tip. (If uncircumcised, pull back foreskin before unrolling condom.)
Unroll condom all the way down to the base of the penis (down to hair).
NOTE: A condom can be put onto a penis that is not fully erect.
Smooth out air bubbles. Make sure condom fits (condoms come in various sizes).

DO USE WITH CONDOMS
Water and saliva
Glycerin
Spermicide
Aloe-9
H-R Lubricating Jelly
K-Y Jelly
Prepair
Probe
AquaLube
Astroglide
ForPlay
Gynol II
Wet
Ramses Personal Spermicide
Touch Personal Lubricant
Eras
Silicone Lubricant
deLube
Liquid silk

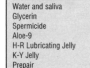

Add WATER-based lubricant to inside and outside of condom if desired.

Condom must be used throughout sex. Afterward, check for breakage/slippage.

After sex: Hold rim of condom and carefully withdraw penis before loss of erection.

Check for breakage. Dispose of condom. If condom breaks, slips, falls off or is not used, use emergency contraception. If not already available, call 888-NOT-2-LATE for Emergency Contraception. Wash areas exposed to body fluids (penis, vagina, etc.) with soap and water.

DO NOT USE WITH LATEX CONDOMS*
Baby oil
Cold creams
Edible oils (olive, peanut, corn, sunflower)
Head and body lotions
Massage oils
Mineral oil
Petroleum jelly
Rubbing alcohol
Shortening (Crisco)
Suntan oil and lotions
Whipped cream
Vegetable oil and cooking oils
Vaginal yeast infection medications in cream or suppository form
• Clindamycin 2% vaginal cream
• Butoconazole cream
• Clotrimazole cream
• Clotrimazole vaginal tablet
• Miconazole vaginal suppository
• Terconazole ointment
• Terconazole cream or vaginal suppository
These lubricants/vaginal products can be used with polyurethane condoms

WHAT IS THE FEMALE CONDOM?

A polyurethane plastic device placed into the vagina. Only one size: 15 centimeters in length and 7 centimeters wide. The flexible and removable inner ring at the closed end is inserted into the vagina as far as possible; the inner ring may be removed or left in place in vagina; the larger outer ring remains outside the vagina. The female condom has a shelf life 3-5 years.

HOW EFFECTIVE ARE FEMALE CONDOMS?

Perfect-use failure rate in first year of use: 5%
Typical-use failure rate in first year of use: 21%
Continuing users after one year: 56%
[Trussell J, Contraceptive Technology, 1998]

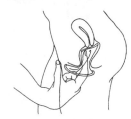

HOW DOES THE FEMALE CONDOM WORK?

Female condoms prevent sperm from entering the vagina.

HOW MUCH DO FEMALE CONDOMS COST?

	Managed-Care Setting	*Public Provider Setting*
Female Condoms	$3.66	$1.25 *[Trussell, 1995; Smith, 1993]*

Retail cost usually $2-3 per condom.

WHAT ARE THE ADVANTAGES OF FEMALE CONDOMS?

Menstrual: Not a hormonal method.
Sexual/psychological:
- Sexual intercourse may be enjoyed more because fear of STIs and pregnancy is decreased
- Transmission of the infection trichomoniasis clearly reduced; probably other infections as well
- Empowers women; provides option to a woman who cannot get a man to use a condom
- If a woman inserts it herself, she can be sure she is protected (no chance of being deceived)
- Can be inserted up to 8 hours before sex; allows spontaneity
- Easier to clean up after sex because condom catches semen
- May be used when man cannot maintain an erection while using male condom
- Although not designed and tested for anal sex, the female condom can be used in the anus for anal sex if the inner ring is taken out

Cancers, tumors, and masses:
- Possible decrease in HPV transmission may reduce risk of cervical cancer

Other:
- In theory, could provide greater STI protection (especially against herpes and HPV) since it covers more of the external genitals
- A portable and immediately effective method
- Breakage is rare
- Available over-the-counter; no medical visit required
- No allergic reactions to latex
- All lubricants are safe (unlike the male condom)
- Polyurethane apparently not damaged by heat
- Good option during breastfeeding
- Protects against pregnancy and infection
- If used consistently and correctly, may reduce the risk for STIs, including HIV *[CDC, 1998]*

WHAT ARE THE DISADVANTAGES OF FEMALE CONDOMS?

Menstrual: Offers none of the potential *benefits* of hormonal contraceptives

Sexual/Psychological:

- Some women do not like the idea of putting fingers or a foreign object into vagina
- Unless put on by the woman in advance, may interrupt sex
- Difficult for some to use properly:
  - Large, bulky and can be difficult for some women to place in vagina
  - Penis must be directed into condom; man may unintentionally place his penis outside the female condom
  - Man must pay attention to possible friction between the condom and his penis (and stop if friction develops)
  - Debatable whether one partner must hold onto outer rim of condom throughout intercourse to be considered "perfect use"
  - Decreased enjoyment of sex from decreased sensation for either partner
  - May cause noise while walking around (if inserted in advance) and during sex
  - Inner ring may cause discomfort; if it does, remove it

Cancers, tumors, and masses: None

Other:

- Clearly less effective than latex male condoms in preventing both pregnancy and STIs
- Hand-washing may need to precede use; hands must be clean to put condom in the vagina
- Purchase, putting on, and disposal may be embarrassing
- Expensive ($3 or more per condom)

WHAT ARE THE RISKS OF FEMALE CONDOMS?

- Infection if left for a long time in vagina; risk of urinary tract infections may increase
- Balance of normal vaginal bacteria may change

WHO CAN USE FEMALE CONDOMS?

- Individuals willing to accept relatively high failure rates
- Those who need a method of protection controlled by the woman
- Individuals only willing to use a single method when infection is a concern
- Those who can use condoms consistently and correctly
- Individuals who have sex in first few weeks after birth when pelvic infection is an important concern (if insertion after birth does not cause pain)
- Pregnant women at risk for infection of any kind

What About Adolescents? The female condom is an appropriate method that provides some protection against pregnancy and infection (best if combined with another method such as pills).

HOW DO I START USING FEMALE CONDOMS?

- Couples need to commit themselves in advance to using condoms every single time
- Woman should practice putting in condom in advance
- Ask your clinician for emergency contraception in advance

WHAT GUIDELINES SHOULD I FOLLOW?

- Do not open the condom package with a pair of scissors; you may cut the condom. Open up the covering of the condom carefully
- When putting the condom into the vagina, avoid tearing the condom or putting a hole in it with fingernails, rings, your teeth, or anything sharp
- Follow the instructions in the package for proper insertion technique
- Remove condom immediately following intercourse, before standing up
- Good for one use only; a new condom must be used for each act of intercourse (studies of re-use of female condom are now under way)
- When the female condom is not used, breaks, or if the penis is placed outside the female condom, use emergency contraception. You may call 1-888-NOT-2-LATE to find the telephone numbers of the 5 nearest providers who will provide emergency contraception
- Drugs and alcohol can greatly reduce consistent and correct use of the female condom
- **Lubricant on the female condom is oil-based and may damage a male condom. If couple wants additional protection against most STIs and against pregnancy, an Avanti male condom or a vaginal spermicide such as contraceptive foam may be used**
- **Do not use the latex male and female condom together; the oil-based lubricant for the Reality female condom can cause breakage of the male condom AND friction can cause condom breakage**

DO I NEED TO CONSULT MY CLINICIAN? ASK YOURSELF:

Following are important questions to help you evaluate your use of the female condom. If you answer "yes" to any question, talk to your clinician to figure out the best solution for you.

☐ Do I have trouble inserting the female condom correctly?

☐ Have I experienced any discomfort from this method?

☐ Are there times when I do not use the female condom?

☐ Do I want or need emergency contraception?

WHAT HAPPENS IF:

I have difficulty inserting? Couples/individuals can learn to use this condom; it takes practice; follow the instructions.

The penis is inserted outside rim? Keep monitoring the position of the penis. Find position for intercourse that does not lead to penis entering outside rim of Reality condom.

WHAT IF I WANT TO GET PREGNANT AFTER USING FEMALE CONDOMS?

- Female condoms can provide excellent protection for future fertility because they can help prevent the infections that cause infertility
- There is no delay in return to fertility

CHAPTER 20

Cervical Cap
www.cervcap.com

WHAT IS A CERVICAL CAP?

The cervical cap is a thimble-shaped latex rubber device. It has a small groove in its inner surface which creates suction to keep cap on cervix. Four sizes are available with internal diameter of 22, 25, 28, 31 centimeters and a woman needs to be fitted. A small amount of spermicide is placed inside the cap before it is placed over the cervix.

cervical cap

HOW EFFECTIVE IS THE CERVICAL CAP?

(Rates include use with spermicide cream or jelly)

	Parous: Women who have given birth	*Nulliparous: Women who have not given birth*
Perfect-use failure rate in first year:	26%	9%
Typical-use failure rate in first year:	40%	20%

[Trussell J, Contraceptive Technology, 1998]

HOW DOES THE CERVICAL CAP WORK?

Stops sperm from going into the cervix and kills sperm when spermicide is used along with the cervical cap. It can be placed in the vagina up to 6 hours before intercourse and should remain at least 6 hours after the last ejaculation and no longer than 48 hours.

HOW MUCH DOES THE CERVICAL CAP COST?

	Managed-Care Setting	*Public Provider Setting*
Cervical cap	$31.00 (lasts 3 years)	$19.00/3 years
Office visit (fitting)	38.00	15.59
Spermicidal jelly (36 applications)	12.00	8.75 *[Trussell, 1995; Smith, 1993]*

WHAT ARE THE ADVANTAGES OF THE CERVICAL CAP?

Menstrual
  • No hormonal side effects
  • Holds back menstrual blood during intercourse. However, this is not generally recommended because of the risk of toxic shock syndrome (see page 7)

Sexual/psychological:
  • Controlled by the woman
  • Can be inserted up to 6 hours before intercourse
  • Can remain in place for multiple acts of intercourse for up to 48 hours
  • May allow spontaneous lovemaking

Cancers, tumors, and masses: None

Other: May reduce risk of cervical infections

WHAT ARE THE DISADVANTAGES OF THE CERVICAL CAP?

Menstrual: Offers none of the potential benefits of hormonal contraceptives

Sexual/psychological:
  • Requires insertion before genital contact, which may reduce spontaneity
  • Some women do not like placing fingers or a foreign body into vagina
  • Odor may develop if cap left in place too long, if not appropriately cleansed, or if used during bacterial vaginosis infection
  • Taste of spermicide may make cunnilingus (oral sex on a woman) unpleasant

Cancers, tumors, and masses
- Labeling requires repeat Pap smear at 3 months after starting because increased risk of cervical changes for first 3 months. No increased risk after one year

Other:
- Lack of protection against some STIs and HIV. Must use condoms if at risk
- Relatively high failure rate
- Requires professional fitting and requires formal (although brief) training
- About 20% of women cannot be fitted
- You must be refitted if you gain or lose 10 or more pounds
- Severe obesity may make it difficult for patient to place cap correctly

WHAT ARE THE RISKS OF THE CERVICAL CAP?
- Urinary tract infections may increase as normal vaginal bacteria changes
- Cervical erosion may occur causing slight vaginal bleeding and/or cervical discomfort. Sometimes a woman's cervix changes size during her menstrual cycle and two different size caps are needed
- No cases of toxic shock syndrome have been reported, but theoretically, the risk is increased, particularly if cap is left in longer than 48 hours or during a woman's period

WHO CAN USE THE CERVICAL CAP?
- Women willing and able to insert the cap before intercourse and take it out later
- Women who have a smooth cervix that can be fit for a cap
- Women with poor muscle tone in the pelvis are better candidates for cap than diaphragm
- Women who are willing to accept a relatively high risk of unintended pregnancy
- Women and partner(s) who have no allergies to latex or spermicides

What About Adolescents? Appropriate option, but fitting and insertion may be difficult for some. Higher failure rates may be a concern for many adolescents.

HOW DO I START THE METHOD?
Fitting:

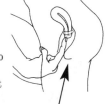

- The cervical cap must be professionally fit by a health care provider
- A pelvic exam is required to judge the size and contour of the cervix, to test for infection and to do a Pap smear
- Your clinician will then insert a cervical cap, starting with the smallest likely size, and will check for proper fit until the correct size is found
- The dome of the cap should completely cover the cervix; the rim of the cap should be tucked snugly and evenly into the areas where the cervix meets the vaginal wall; make a sweep with your finger around the entire cervix to make sure there are no gaps
- The cap should not move on the cervix during the fitting exam or during regular use
- If a gap is found, see if the rim can be pulled away with direct pressure (if yes, the cap is probably too big and a smaller size should be tried)
- After the cap has been in place for at least a minute, check the suction by pinching the excess rubber on the dome between the tips of two fingers and tugging. The dome should dimple, but not collapse
- You should not be able to dislodge the cap by gently tugging or pulling on it with one or two fingers from several angles
- After the cap is successfully fit, it is removed by pushing the rim away from the cervix with one or two fingers to break the suction and then gently pulling the cap out of the vagina
- It is a good idea to try putting the cervical cap in yourself in front of your clinician to make sure you are comfortable inserting and removing it
- It is recommended for you to get emergency contraception in advance in case you need it—ask your clinician

WHAT GUIDELINES DO I NEED TO FOLLOW?
- *To put the cervical cap in:* fill the bottom 1/3 of the cap with spermicide and put the cap in place before intercourse
- Test the fit to ensure cervix is covered, with no gaps between the cervix and the cap; after suction develops for about 1 minute, the device should not dislodge with pressure
- Keep the cap in place for 6 hours after last intercourse
- If you have sex more than once, there is no need to add more spermicide but you need to make sure the cap is still in correct position before next act of intercourse
- Do not leave the cap in place for more than 48 hours, if you have an infection, or during your period because it increases your risk of toxic shock syndrome (see page 7)
- Do not expose the cap to oil-based products such as vaseline, baby oil, yeast infection creams and oil-based antibiotic creams (see page 49)
- If cap dislodges, emergency contraception is available
- Use a backup method the first few times until you are confident in your use of the cap
- Combining the cap and the male condom or the female condom can increase protection against pregnancy and infection
- Drug and alcohol use can reduce the effectiveness of the cervical cap. Being drunk or using other drugs increases the risk of making a mistake
- The FDA recommends a follow-up Pap smear after 3 months
- Do not use the cap for at least 2 or 3 days before routine gynecological exams because it can interfere with the Pap smear. Use a different method if needed

TO REMOVE THE CERVICAL CAP:
- Cap should not be removed until 6 hours after last ejaculation, but before 48 hours
- Insert a finger into the vagina until you feel the rim of the cap
- Press the cap rim until the seal against the cervix is broken; then tilt the cap off the cervix
- Hook finger around the rim and pull it sideways out of the vagina
- The device must be washed, rinsed, dried and stored in a cool, dark and dry location
- Rinsing in Listerine® can prevent odors that occasionally occur

DO I NEED TO CONSULT MY CLINICIAN? ASK YOURSELF:
Following are important questions to help you evaluate your use of the cervical cap. If you answer "yes" to any question, talk to your clinician to figure out the best solution for you.
- ☐ Am I or is my partner experiencing any tenderness or irritation?
- ☐ Is the odor of the cap a problem?
- ☐ Are there times when I do not use the female condom?
- ☐ Would I like to have emergency contraception with me?

WHAT HAPPENS IF:
I have spotting or cervical tenderness? Stop use to allow healing. Contact your clinician to get refit with a larger cap.

My cap smells bad? Listerine soaks may help. You may also shorten the time the cap is left in place, or replace the cap.

I fail to use it correctly? Use emergency contraception. If it is not already available, call 1-888-NOT-2-LATE or 1-888-PREVEN2.

WHAT HAPPENS IF I WANT TO GET PREGNANT AFTER USING THE CERVICAL CAP?
The cervical cap has no adverse effects on fertility; fertility returns immediately.

WHAT IS THE DIAPHRAGM?

Rubber dome-shaped device filled with spermicide that is placed inside vagina to cover cervix. Four types of diaphragms are available. You must be fitted by a clinician:

- *Arcing spring:* puts even pressure around its rim to cover the cervix
- *Coil spring:* most appropriate for women with a deep pubic arch or average vaginal muscle tone
- *Flat spring:* most appropriate for women with a shallow pubic arch or strong vaginal muscle tone
- *Wide seal:* extends inward from the rim to contain the spermicide

HOW EFFECTIVE IS THE DIAPHRAGM?

Perfect-use failure rate in first year: 6%
Typical-use failure rate in first year: 20%
[Trussell J, Contraceptive Technology, 1998]

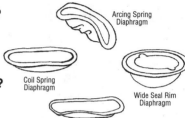

Arcing Spring Diaphragm

Coil Spring Diaphragm

Wide Seal Rim Diaphragm

Flat Spring Diaphragm

HOW DOES THE DIAPHRAGM WORK?

It prevents sperm from going into the cervix and the spermicide used with it kills sperm.

HOW MUCH DOES THE DIAPHRAGM COST?

	Managed-Care Setting	*Public Provider Setting*
Device	$18.00 (lasts 3 years)	$15.00 (lasts 3 years)
Office Visit (device fitting)	38.00	15.59
Spermicidal Jelly	12.00	8.75
(12 applications)		[Trussell, 1995; Smith, 1993]

WHAT ARE THE ADVANTAGES OF THE DIAPHRAGM?

Menstrual: No hormonal side effects
Sexual/psychological:

- Controlled by the woman
- May be inserted before intercourse (within 6 hrs)
- May allow spontaneous lovemaking

Cancers, tumors, and masses: None (except perhaps cervical cancer by decreasing risk for HPV infection, but this has not been proven)
Other:

- Reduces risk for cervical infections, including gonorrhea, chlamydia, human papilloma virus (HPV), and pelvic inflammatory disease (PID)
- Is used only with intercourse
- May be used during breastfeeding after vagina and cervix have returned to non-pregnant shape

WHAT ARE THE DISADVANTAGES OF THE DIAPHRAGM?

Menstrual: Offers none of the potential benefits of hormonal contraceptives

Sexual/psychological:
- Requires placement before genital contact which may interrupt spontaneity of lovemaking
- Taste of spermicide may discourage oral sex
- Some women dislike placing fingers or a foreign object into vagina

Cancer, tumors, and masses: None

Other:
- Requires professional fitting; severe obesity may make fitting difficult
- May not be feasible for women with pelvic relaxation (poor muscle tone)
- Relatively high failure rates
- Requires brief, formal training and some coordination to insert and remove
- May develop odor if not properly cleansed

WHAT ARE THE RISKS OF THE DIAPHRAGM?

- May increase risk of urinary tract infection, due to an increase in certain bacteria in the vagina
- May increase risk of toxic shock syndrome (TSS), especially if used for long periods of time or during your period (see page 6)
- Large, poorly fitted diaphragm may cause vaginal irritation
- May become messy with multiple acts of intercourse

WHO CAN USE THE DIAPHRAGM?

- Women/couples who can predict when intercourse will occur
- Highly motivated women/couples willing to use it every time they have intercourse
- Women/couples who are willing to accept a higher risk of pregnancy

What About Adolescents: Appropriate, if taught to use consistently and correctly; requires discipline. Higher failure rate may be a concern for many adolescents.

HOW DO I START THE METHOD?

- Each woman needs to be fitted
- A pelvic examination will rule out any vaginal/cervical problems
- Using fingers, your clinician will measure your vagina to select the size of the diaphragm and to place a fitting diaphragm in the vagina
- You will walk around for a while in your clinician's office to test its long-term comfort
- It is a good idea to have your clinician check your ability to insert and remove diaphragm
- It is good to use a backup method for the first few times to make sure you can use it correctly
- Get emergency contraception in advance— ask your clinician

WHAT GUIDELINES DO I NEED TO FOLLOW?

- Fill inner surface of diaphragm 2/3's full with 2 teaspoons of spermicide before insertion. Insert before genital contact but no longer than 6 hours before intercourse. It can remain in place for up to 24 hours
- Squeeze the ring together with your thumb and index finger. Insert the diaphragm into your vagina using your index finger. The diaphragm should fit snugly over the cervix

Risk of pregnancy increases when a spermicide is not used

- Before each act of intercourse, reconfirm correct placement. If you wish to have intercourse again, add more spermicide into the vagina using the applicator that comes with the spermicide but do not remove the diaphragm
- Leave in place for at least 6 hours after the last act of intercourse
- Avoid using any oil-based vaginal products such as Vaseline, yeast infection creams or some antibiotic creams (see list of products that are UNSAFE to use with latex condoms, page 49)
- After removal, clean with soap and water, rinse, dry, and store in the case in a cool, clean, dry, dark area
- Check regularly for any stiffness, holes, cracks, or other defects by holding it up to light or putting it in water to watch for bubbles
- Have it checked each year by a clinician. Replace at least every 3 years. Recheck for correct fit whenever there is a 20% weight loss or gain, and after each pregnancy
- Combine diaphragm with male condoms to reduce pregnancy and STI risk
- Drug and alcohol use can reduce the effectiveness of the diaphragm. Being drunk or high increases the risk of making a mistake
- If diaphragm dislodges or is not used properly, use emergency contraception

DO I NEED TO CONSULT MY CLINICIAN? ASK YOURSELF:

Following are important questions to help you evaluate your use of the diaphragm. If you answer "yes" to any question, talk to your clinician to figure out the best solution for you.

☐ Do I get bladder infections often?
☐ Have I or has my partner had an allergic reaction (burning or itching)?
☐ Are there times when I do not use the diaphragm?
☐ Are there times when I do not apply a spermicide before insertion?
☐ Do I want emergency contraception to have with me in case of an accident?

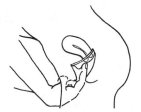

Reconfirm correct placement by feeling the cervix through the diaphragm

WHAT HAPPENS IF:

I am prone to cystitis? Urinate after sex to reduce growth of vaginal bacteria in bladder.

I am allergic to latex? Stop use and discuss alternatives with your clinician.

My diaphragm smells bad? Listerine soaks may help. You may also shorten the time the diaphragm is left in place, or replace the diaphragm.

WHAT IF I WANT TO GET PREGNANT AFTER USING THE DIAPHRAGM?

- No adverse effects on fertility
- Protects fertility by reducing risk of pelvic inflammatory disease

CHAPTER 22

Spermicides and Contraceptive Sponge

WHAT ARE SPERMICIDES?
In the USA, octoxynol-9 (O-9) and nonoxynol-9 (N-9) are available over the counter. In addition to these spermicides, people in other parts of the world use menfegol, benzalkonium chloride, sodium docusate, and chlorhexidine. Spermicides come in the form of vaginal creams, films, foams, gels, suppositories, tablets, and sponges.

HOW DO SPERMICIDES WORK?
Perfect-use failure rate in first year: 6%
Typical-use failure rate in first year: 26%   *[Trussell J, Contraceptive Technology, 1998]*

HOW DO SPERMICIDES WORK?
As barriers, they block sperm from entering the cervix. As chemicals, they attack the sperm's tail and body, both reducing mobility, and decreasing nourishment.

HOW MUCH DO SPERMICIDES COST?
Varies from state to state; national averages are:

Creams/Gels	$10.08 for 8 oz
Film (VCF) (see figure)	$12.26 for 12
Foam	$11.23 for 0.6 oz
Suppositories/Tabs	$12.79 for 18 inserts

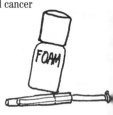
vaginal film

WHAT ARE THE ADVANTAGES OF SPERMICIDES?
Menstrual: No hormonal side effects or complications
Sexual/psychological:
  • Lubrication, in the case of foam, may heighten satisfaction in both partners
  • Ease in applying (for some women) before or during intercourse
  • Either partner can purchase and apply
  • May be used by woman without partner knowing
Cancers, tumors, and masses:
  • Possible decrease in HPV transmission may reduce risk of cervical cancer
Other:
  • Available over the counter; does not require visit to a clinician
  • Inexpensive
  • Sporadic use/stopping possible
  • Can use during breastfeeding
  • Makes cervical cap and diaphragm more effective
  • Serves as immediate back-up if condom should break or slip

WHAT ARE THE DISADVANTAGES OF SPERMICIDES?
Menstrual:
  • Offers none of the potential benefits of hormonal contraceptives
Sexual/psychological:
  • At least one partner must feel comfortable inserting fingers into vagina
  • Insertion is not easy for some couples
  • Some methods (foam) become "messy" during intercourse

- Minimal, if any, protection against STIs/HIV
- Possible vaginal, oral, and anal irritation can interrupt or stop sex
- Taste may be unpleasant

Cancers, tumors, and masses: None

Other:
- People have confused fruit jelly (e.g., grape jelly) for spermicidal "jelly"
- People attempt to use cosmetics or hair products containing non-spermicidal octoxynols and nonoxynols (nonoxynol 4, 10, 12, and 14) instead of nonoxynol-9

WHAT ARE THE RISKS OF SPERMICIDES?
- Allergic reactions in women and men could decrease use
- Might increase likelihood of STIs and UTIs through irritation of vaginal lining and by causing an imbalance in normal vaginal bacteria
- Reported infection protection might make someone less likely to use condoms for STI protection (false sense of security)

WHO CAN USE SPERMICIDES?
- Any woman who has no prior allergy or reaction to spermicides, is aware of pros and cons, and knows the signs of allergy or irritation
- Any woman who will use a female condom or whose male partner will use a condom as a secondary method
- Women who are willing to accept a higher risk of pregnancy

What About Adolescents? Appropriate method. However, there is no documented effectiveness against HIV and, used alone, spermicides are less effective than condoms in preventing other STIs. Simultaneous use of condoms may reduce risk of HIV/STIs.

HOW DO I START THE METHOD?
- Except in cases where the woman, or partner, is pregnant, allergic to, or irritated by spermicides, it is OK to start these methods at any time
- Get emergency contraception in advance—ask your clinician

WHAT GUIDELINES DO I NEED TO FOLLOW?
- Before and after applying spermicide, inserting person should wash and dry hands
- Spermicide should not be expired and package should have no defects
- Spermicide is most effective near the cervical opening
- Use more spermicide for each act of intercourse
- Water (bathing or douching) within 6 hours after insertion or after intercourse makes spermicides less effective; reapply before next intercourse
- Keep spermicides in cool, dry places; tablets or foam can tolerate heat; film melts at 98.6° F (body temperature)
- Drugs and alcohol can greatly reduce the effectiveness of spermicides. Being drunk or using other drugs increases the risk of making a mistake

Creams/foams/gels
- Apply less than 1 hour before intercourse. May drip out of vagina if inserted more than 1 hour in advance. With foam, shake canister vigorously. Fill plastic applicator with spermicide. Insert applicator deeply into vagina and push plunger in (similar to tampon insertion)

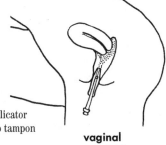
vaginal spermicide

Film, suppositories and tablets
- Insert less than 1 hour, but at least 15 minutes before intercourse; with film, fold the sheet in half and then half again (this aids insertion). Using fingers or an applicator, the inserting partner places the spermicide suppository, tablet, or film deeply in the vagina, as near to the cervix as possible

DO I NEED TO CONSULT MY CLINICIAN? ASK YOURSELF:

Following are important questions to help you evaluate your use of spermicides. If you answer "yes" to any question, talk to your clinician to figure out the best solution for you.

☐ Have I or my partner(s) experienced any rash or discomfort?
☐ Have I changed partners since beginning spermicides?
☐ Have I had sex using spermicide alone?
☐ Would I like emergency contraception to have in case of an accident?

WHAT HAPPENS IF:

I have dermatitis (itching and irritation)? Stop using spermicides and use a secondary method. If you have been using spermicide as a lubricant, you can use instead a water-based or silicon-based lubricant without nonoxynol-9 or octoxynol-9.

I changed sex partners? It is a good idea for you and your new partner to be tested for infections and to use condoms to prevent infections.

I use spermicide alone? If you are still at risk for infection, use a backup method such as condoms to increase protection.

WHAT HAPPENS IF I WANT TO GET PREGNANT AFTER USING SPERMICIDES?

Fertility returns immediately.

CONTRACEPTIVE SPONGE
Late Breaking News!

For thousands of years women have placed sponges with a variety of spermicides into the vagina. The Today Contraceptive Sponge (Elaine's favorite method from *Seinfield*) will soon be back on pharmacy shelves in the United States. This is exciting news because women who liked the sponge were very loyal to it. It was taken off the market in 1995 because the company that produced it decided it was too costly to update its manufacturing facility.

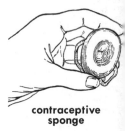

contraceptive sponge

WHAT IS THE CONTRACEPTIVE SPONGE?

A small piece of polyurethane foam containing spermicide that is inserted in the vagina to cover the cervix.

HOW EFFECTIVE IS THE SPONGE? *[Trussell, 1998]*

Perfect-use failure rate in first year of use in women who have had a baby: 20%
Typical-use failure rate in first year of use in women who have had a baby: 40%

Perfect-use failure rate in first year of use in women who have never had a baby: 9%
Typical-use failure rate in first year of use in women who have never had a baby: 20%

These rates are different because after a woman has a baby, her cervix changes, making the sponge fit less accurately.

HOW DOES THE SPONGE WORK?

The sponge itself blocks sperm from going into the cervix and the spermicide in the sponge kills or immobilizes sperm.

HOW MUCH DOES THE SPONGE COST?

Unknown until it reappears in drug stores.

WHAT ARE THE ADVANTAGES OF THE SPONGE?

Menstrual: No hormonal side effects

Sexual/psychological:

- May be inserted up to 2 hours before intercourse and may be left in up to 12 hours after
- If you do not take the sponge out, you do not need a new sponge each time you have intercourse (within the 12 hours)

Cancers, tumors, masses: None

Other:

- May protect against some infections (chlamydia and gonorrhea)
- You do not need a prescription to get the sponge
- Can use during breastfeeding
- Serves as immediate backup if condom breaks or slips

WHAT ARE THE DISADVANTAGES OF THE SPONGE?

Menstrual: None of the potential benefits of hormonal contraceptives

Sexual/psychological:

- Either partner must feel comfortable inserting fingers and a foreign object into vagina
- During intercourse, your partner might be able to feel the sponge, or it might slip out

Cancers, tumors, masses: None

Other:

- Cannot be used if woman or man is allergic to nonoxynol-9 or if woman has had toxic shock syndrome (TSS)
- Does not protect against many infections, including HIV
- Changes in vaginal discharge are possible and the sponge might increase risk of yeast infections

WHAT GUIDELINES SHOULD I FOLLOW?

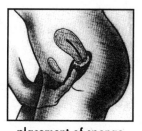

placement of sponge

- Insert the sponge into the vagina just before or up to 2 hours before intercourse
- Leave in place for at least 6-8 hours and no longer than 12 hours after sex
- Do not leave the sponge in the vagina for more than 24 hours total. Doing so increases your risk of toxic shock syndrome (see page 6)
- Remove sponge by pulling on a ribbon attached to one side
- Discard the sponge after use
- Stop using immediately and contact your clinician if you are unable to remove the sponge, get soreness in the vagina, a rash in the genital area, a lot of foul-smelling or itchy discharge, severe abdominal pain, and/or fever or chills for no reason
- Drugs or alcohol can greatly reduce the effectiveness of the sponge. Being drunk or high increases the risk of making a mistake

Withdrawal (Coitus Interruptus)

WHAT IS WITHDRAWAL?
Withdrawal is when a man removes his penis completely from the vagina before he ejaculates (comes). Coitus (in the term "coitus interruptus") is the medical term for penile-vaginal sexual intercourse.

HOW EFFECTIVE IS WITHDRAWAL?
Perfect-use failure rate in first year: 4%
Typical-use failure rate in first year: 19%
[Trussell J, Contraceptive Technology, 1998]

HOW DOES WITHDRAWAL WORK?
Withdrawal before ejaculation reduces or stops sperm from going into vagina. NOTE: Preejaculatory fluid (precum) can contain sperm, making conception possible, and may transmit HIV and other STIs.

HOW MUCH DOES WITHDRAWAL COST? Nothing—it's free

WHAT ARE THE ADVANTAGES OF WITHDRAWAL?
Menstrual: Non-hormonal; no hormonal side effects or complications
Sexual/psychological:
  - No barrier methods are needed and abstinence avoided
  - Readily available method which encourages male involvement
  - May introduce variety into sexual relationship
  - May increase spontaneity of sex
  - After practice, may increase a man's understanding and awareness of his sexual response cycle
Cancers, tumors, and masses: None
Other: Surprisingly effective if used correctly

WHAT ARE THE DISADVANTAGES OF WITHDRAWAL?
Menstrual: Offers none of the potential benefits of hormonal contraceptives
Sexual/psychological
  - Individuals with sexual dysfunction such as premature ejaculation or unpredictable ejaculation may not be able to use (see chapter 5)
  - Man's instruction and cooperation is needed; requires a great deal of trust
  - May reduce sexual pleasure of woman and intensity of orgasm of man
  - Encourages "spectatoring," or observing and analyzing what is happening during sex rather than enjoying it
  - Increased fear of pregnancy and infection may decrease enjoyment of sex
Cancers, tumors, and masses: No impact
Other: Relatively high failure rate among typical users and does not protect adequately against infection

WHAT ARE THE RISKS OF WITHDRAWAL? No protection against infections.

IS WITHDRAWAL THE RIGHT METHOD FOR ME?

1. Is the man unable to predict ejaculation in time to withdraw penis completely from vagina and vaginal opening?

☐ No   ☐ Yes   If yes, withdrawal may not be a good method for you.

2. Does the man have premature ejaculation?

☐ No   ☐ Yes   If yes, withdrawal will not be as effective. You may want to consider another method.

3. Do you or your partner have a sexually transmitted infection or are you at risk for infection?

☐ No   ☐ Yes   If yes, withdrawal does not provide adequate protection against infection. Consider another method.

WHO CAN USE WITHDRAWAL?

• Individuals who are able to communicate during sex
• Disciplined men who are aware of their sexual response and who can stop thrusting
• Individuals without religious or cultural rules against withdrawal
• Individuals willing to accept higher risk of pregnancy

What About Adolescents? Tend not to use it consistently. Use of condoms is better for protection against pregnancy and infections, however, withdrawal is better than no pregnancy protection at all.

HOW DO I START THE METHOD?

• Can begin at any time
• You can get emergency contraception in advance

WHAT GUIDELINES DO I NEED TO FOLLOW?

• Practice withdrawal using a backup method, until both partners master withdrawal
• Wipe penis clean of the pre-ejaculation fluid before intercourse
• Use sexual positions that reduce deep vaginal penetration: 1) male putting the penis in part way in the male-on-top position; 2) the female-on-top position; and 3) side-by-side (spooning)
• Drugs or alcohol can greatly reduce the effectiveness of withdrawal. Being drunk or high increases the risk of making a mistake
• Use emergency contraception if withdrawal fails

DO I NEED TO CONSULT MY CLINICIAN? ASK YOURSELF:

Following are important questions to help you evaluate your use of withdrawal. If you answer "yes" to any question, talk to your clinician to figure out the best solution for you.

☐ Does my partner ever ejaculate or begin to ejaculate before withdrawing his penis?

WHAT HAPPENS IF:

The man fails to withdraw? If withdrawal does not happen every time, you can use emergency contraception.

WHAT IF I WANT TO GET PREGNANT AFTER USING WITHDRAWAL?

No direct effect on fertility, but withdrawal may put a woman at risk of sexually transmitted infections that can lead to infertility.

Is it an Emergency?

We had the greatest date—a romantic dinner, a moonlight walk under the stars, and drinks back at her apartment. I didn't expect to have sex with her but things started really getting hot. Before I knew it we were naked in my bed and we had intercourse. It only lasted a few minutes before we both decided to stop, but there was preejaculatory fluid and now I'm really worried about the risk of her being pregnant...

* * * * *

We have two children and have decided not to have any more. We use condoms every time during sex and have never experienced a problem. This morning, however, the condom broke during our lovemaking. It didn't feel any different but when we took it off, we found a little tear near the tip...

* * * * *

I am so confused right now. Last night I was hanging out in my dorm room with this guy I have been friends with for the past 6 months. There has always been sexual tension between us and last night we finally started to act on it. He got really aggressive, though, and I feel like he really coerced, even forced, me into having sex with him. The worst part is that we didn't even use any protection. I don't know what I would do if I were pregnant...

* * * * *

My partner has been taking birth control pills for about 4 years and is really good about taking them every day at the same time. However, this month she forgot to take the first pill in the new cycle. We are scared that she might be pregnant because we had sex the night before...

Do any of these situations sound familiar? If so, there is something you can do about it. Taking emergency contraception as soon as possible (and within 72 hours) after unprotected sex can help prevent unintended pregnancy. Call 1-888-NOT-2-LATE to get the name of a clinician near you who will prescribe emergency contraception.

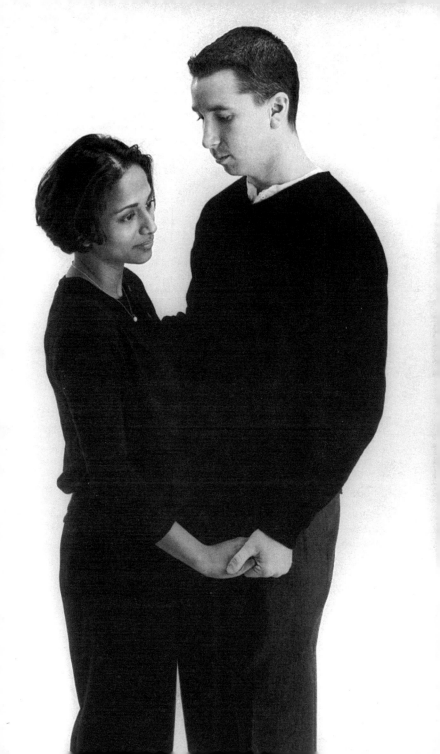

WHY IS EMERGENCY CONTRACEPTION IMPORTANT?

Emergency contraception is pregnancy prevention after unprotected sex, suspected contraceptive failure, or rape. Making emergency contraception widely available is one of the most important steps that we can take to reduce the unacceptable level of unintended pregnancy in the United States. There are 3 million unintended pregnancies each year; half of all pregnancies are unintended. Making emergency contraception widely available could cut the number of unintended pregnancies in half and reduce the need for abortion.

WHAT ARE THE CURRENTLY AVAILABLE EMERGENCY CONTRACEPTIVE OPTIONS?

- Progestin-only pills (POPs) as emergency contraception (PLAN B: 1 + 1 pill 12 hours later; Ovrette: 20 pills then 20 pills 12 hours later per dose). Take as soon as possible, within 72 hours. PLAN B is safe; so safe that in France, it is available over-the-counter without a prescription. See dedication to read about the woman who brought PLAN B to women in the U.S., Dr. Sharon Camp. In the U.S., PLAN B is currently available with a prescription only
- Combined oral contraceptive pills (COCs) as emergency contraception (Preven: 2+2 pills 12 hours later; plus other options). Take as soon as possible, within 72 hours. Preven is available in the U.S. with a prescription only
- Copper T 380-A IUD insertion for up to 5-8 days after unprotected sex
- RU-486 (mifepristone) **within 5 days** of unprotected intercourse is emergency contraception, not an abortion (not currently available in the U.S.). RU-486 as emergency contraception uses a much lower dose than when it is used to perform an abortion

WHAT ARE BASICS ABOUT EMERGENCY CONTRACEPTION?

- For emergency contraception to be most effective, it should begin as soon as possible (within 72 hours after unprotected sex for pills and wiht 5 days for IUD). Any delay lowers the effectiveness, making it important to have emergency contraception on hand in case it is needed
- Each approach available today in the United States reduces risk of pregnancy; *it does not cause an abortion.* Abortion stops pregnancy after the fertilized egg implants in the uterus (the medical definition of pregnancy); emergency contraception will not disrupt an established pregnancy
- Immediately after getting emergency contraception you need to start ongoing contraception

For more information and phone numbers of clinicians in your telephone area code, check out www.opr.princeton.edu, www.PREVEN.com, or www.go2planB.com or call **1-888-NOT-2-LATE. 1-888-PREVEN2 provides information but NOT phone numbers of clinicians.**

Although emergency contraceptive pills prevent most of the pregnancies which follow a single act of intercourse, they are no where near as effective as ongoing contraceptives. The failure rates for ongoing contraceptive methods are for an entire year (see page 35) during which a woman usually has many acts of intercourse during most months of the year.

Overview of emergency contraceptive methods currently available in the USA. You can get emergency contraception in advance.

	Progestin-Only Pills (POPs)	Combined Oral Contraceptives (COCs)	Copper IUD
Timing after intercourse	Up to 72 hours; the sooner the better	Up to 72 hours; the sooner the better	Up to 5 days, maybe longer*
Pregnancies per 100 women	1.1% *[WHO, 1998]*	3.2%	0.1%
Most important advantage	Less nausea (23.1%) or vomiting (5.6%) than with combined pills	Many different COCs available: Preven, Ovral and 8 others	May be inserted as long as 5-8 days after unprotected sex (see page 76) Most effective method
Most important disadvantage	Previously had to take 20 Ovrette pills twice (But now with PLAN B, 1 pill twice)	Nausea (50%) or vomiting (20%) without anti-nausea drugs	Some women poor candidates; don't want an IUD; expensive
Side effects	Nausea and vomiting but lower rates	Nausea and vomiting	Pain, bleeding, risk of infection
Avoid use for these reasons	Pregnancy or you suspect you are pregnant	Pregnancy; current migraine with focal neurological symptoms; history of blood clots in the legs or lungs	Pregnancy; other IUD precautions (see page 83)

*The Copper T 380-A IUD may be inserted up to the time of implantation (about 5 days after ovulation) to prevent pregnancy. Thus, if you had unprotected intercourse 3 days before ovulation in that cycle, the IUD could be inserted up to 8 days after intercourse to prevent pregnancy.

IMPORTANT NOTES ON PROGESTIN–ONLY PILLS (POPs) AS EMERGENCY CONTRACEPTION

- Total amount of hormone taken is very small (.75 milligrams of levonorgestrel), but it used to be that the number of pills you had to take was large. Now all the hormone a woman must take is available in a single pill, which a woman takes and then takes again in 12 hours. This is called "PLAN B." It is available through most Planned Parenthood clinics now and soon (or even by the time you read this book) will be in pharmacies
- PLAN B is LESS expensive than other emergency contraceptive options. Using Ovrette, the other way to use progestin-only pills as emergency contraception, is more expensive than using combined pills as emergency contraception
- Only 1.1% of 967 women using progestin-only pills as emergency contraception became pregnant in a World Health Organization study *[WHO, 1998]*
- Stops or delays ovulation, preventing fertilization; may change uterine lining, preventing implantation; may change movement of sperm or egg
- No increased risk for blood clots
- Probably a better option than combined pills for women who have had deep vein thrombosis (severe blood clots in the legs) or blood clots in the lungs
- Nausea (23.1%) and vomiting (5.6%) are less common in women using progestin-only pills than combined pills
- May change amount, timing and length of next menstrual period
- Other possible side effects: breast tenderness, fatigue, headache, abdominal pain, and dizziness
- Possibility of ectopic pregnancy if treatment fails (but no increased risk)
- Fertility returns after next period

EMERGENCY CONTRACEPTIVE PILLS, OFTEN CALLED ECPs:

WHAT ARE EMERGENCY CONTRACEPTIVE PILLS (ECPS)?

Two large doses of progestin-only pills or combined oral contraceptive pills (with the hormone norgestrel or levonorgestrel) taken as soon as possible after unprotected intercourse. First dose needs to be taken within 72 hours after unprotected sex, with the second dose 12 hours later. They are more effective the earlier they are taken, but may be somewhat effective even if the first dose is taken after 72 hours. Taking more than the number of pills you are supposed to is not helpful. PLAN B and the PREVEN™ kit are the only currently available products with specific instructions for the user included.

HOW EFFECTIVE ARE ORAL CONTRACEPTIVES AS EMERGENCY CONTRACEPTIVE PILLS?

- If each of 100 women has a single act of unprotected intercourse on one of the days in the middle 2 weeks of the cycle and then take ECPs, only 1%-3% will become pregnant (1.1% using POPs and 3.2% using COCs versus about 8% if no emergency contraception is used)
- A recent article suggests that COCs prevent only about 57% of pregnancies that would otherwise have occurred and that POPs prevent 85% of pregnancies that would otherwise have occurred *[WHO, 1998]*
- If a woman is pregnant, there is no known harm to the woman, the course of the pregnancy, or the fetus if combined or progestin-only pills are used

HOW DO ORAL CONTRACEPTIVES WORK AS EMERGENCY CONTRACEPTION?

If taken before ovulation, ECPs may stop normal egg growth, which prevents ovulation, delays ovulation or decreases hormone production. If taken after ovulation, they may have an effect on the growth of the lining of the uterus thus preventing implantation. They may also affect the movement of sperm or egg in ways that interfere with fertilization.

HOW MUCH DO EMERGENCY CONTRACEPTIVE PILLS COST?

- The PREVEN™ kit: Pills plus pregnancy test: $20-$25 at pharmacies. Almost all public family planning clinics do a pregnancy test before giving emergency contraception. Publically supported clinics can buy the PREVEN™ kit at prices less than $5 per kit. If the pregnancy test in the PREVEN™ kit is not used before taking pills, it may be used several weeks later if you are late for your period.
- NOTE: Some pharmacies will not fill emergency contraception prescriptions because they believe it is abortion. Ask your clinician which pharmacies will fill your prescription before you go
- One cycle of pills may vary from a few dollars to more than $50. Ovral tends to be more expensive than other combined pills and is no longer carried in all drug stores. Two cycles of Ovrette may cost $60 or more
- The cost before getting pills varies from nothing (if free at a clinic) to the cost of a phone call to the cost of a full exam and pregnancy test
- PLAN B is not available in all pharmacies as of May 2000. The cost of PLAN B in pharmacies and in bulk sales will probably be about the same as the PREVEN kit

WHAT ARE THE ADVANTAGES OF EMERGENCY CONTRACEPTIVE PILLS?

Menstrual: None

Sexual/psychological:

- Gives you the opportunity to prevent pregnancy after forced intercourse, a mistake, or a condom breakage
- Offers the option of pregnancy prevention if you suspect you are at risk (instead of waiting to find out)
- The process of getting emergency contraception may lead you to start ongoing contraception

Cancers, tumors, and masses: None

Other:

- No increased risk for birth defects if pills are taken by an already pregnant woman
- **It is not dangerous to use emergency contraceptive pills more than once,** but it is necessary to find an on-going method of contraception that you will use consistently and correctly. If emergency contraception is needed more than once in the same menstrual cycle, it is not dangerous for a woman

WHAT ARE THE DISADVANTAGES OF EMERGENCY CONTRACEPTIVE PILLS?

Menstrual:

- Your next period may be early (especially if pills are taken before ovulation), on time, or late
- About 10%-15% of women have minor changes in their periods (heavier, lighter, earlier, or later)

Sexual/psychological:

- If you are opposed to emergency contraceptive methods that prevent implantation of a fertilized egg, it is important to know that taking emergency contraceptive pills before ovulation can prevent fertilization by preventing or delaying ovulation

Cancers, tumors, and masses: None

Other:

- Nausea in 50% of women and vomiting in 5-25% are the major problems
- Breast tenderness, fatigue, headache, abdominal pain and dizziness
- No protection against sexually transmitted infections; you may need to be treated for infection
- There is a possibility of ectopic pregnancy if pills fail (ECPs prevent some, but not all ectopics)

WHAT ARE THE RISKS OF USING PILLS AS EMERGENCY CONTRACEPTION?

Several cases of deep vein thrombosis (severe blood clots) have been reported from using combined pills as emergency contraception. No serious complications were reported in the collaborative World Health Organization study of progestin-only pills used as emergency contraceptives *[WHO, 1998]*.

WHO CAN USE EMERGENCY CONTRACEPTIVE PILLS?

- Women who were forced to have intercourse against their will
- Women who failed to use contraception, had a partner who failed to use contraception, or had a condom break; women who used a diaphragm without spermicide, had an IUD that expelled, missed pills or started a package of pills late, or used withdrawal incorrectly
- Almost all women can use them, including most women with precautions against regular use of combined pills (e.g., smokers over 35; women who have had breast cancer)
- Smokers of all ages
- Women who have never had a pelvic exam
- Women in any phase of the menstrual cycle (not just for unprotected intercourse at midcycle)
- If in doubt, ask your clinician about emergency contraception or call 1-888-NOT-2-LATE

What About Adolescents? Appropriate emergency option; but they should also be encouraged to use a more effective, ongoing method for birth control and condoms for protection against infection.

ARE EMERGENCY CONTRACEPTIVE PILLS THE RIGHT METHOD FOR ME?

1. Do you have a proven history of deep vein thrombosis (severe blood clots in the legs) or blood clots in the lungs?

☐ No   ☐ Yes   If yes, use progestin-only pills (PLAN B or Ovrette) or Copper T 380-A instead of combined pills.

2. Have you had severe nausea/vomiting from using combined pills in the past?

☐ No   ☐ Yes   If yes, use progestin-only pills (PLAN B or Ovrette) or Copper T 380-A. It is probably as effective to place emergency contraceptive pills in the vagina if vomiting occurs from taking the hormones in birth control pills.

3. Are you pregnant?

☐ No   ☐ Yes   If yes, avoid all pills as emergency contraception; they will NOT damage the fetus, but they are not effective.

HOW DO I START THE METHOD? As soon as possible!

- Ask your clinician about getting emergency contraception in advance. If you have emergency contraceptive pills in your medicine chest, you can use them immediately should an emergency occur. Take ECPs as soon as possible. Each 12 hour delay in taking emergency contraceptive pills lowers their effectiveness
- Not currently available without a prescription except in the state of Washington where over 150 pharmacies can and do provide ECPs to women without a prescription
- Call emergency contraception hotline number 1-888- NOT- 2-LATE to get the phone numbers of 5 clinics or clinicians near you who will provide ECPs. It has excellent information in English and Spanish and up-to-date information on PLAN B
- Many clinicians will prescribe emergency contraception without a pelvic exam
- Many clinicians will prescribe emergency contraception over the telephone
- A pregnancy test may be performed, but emergency contraception is often prescribed without one. If pills from PREVEN™ package are used without the pregnancy test, the pregnancy test may be used several weeks later if your period is late
- If you have a history of severe blood clots in the legs or blood clots in the lungs, you should use progestin-only pills (PLAN B or Ovrette) instead of combined pills
- If you have migraine headaches with neurological symptoms at the present time, you should take progestin-only pills (PLAN B or Ovrette) instead of combined pills
- If you think you might be pregnant, you should take a pregnancy test before using emergency contraception
- Even if you do not have intercourse often, you should **not** count on emergency contraception as on-going contraception because it is not as effective as other methods and tends to cause nausea and vomiting and irregular menstrual cycles. Repeated use is also expensive
- If you use emergency contraception after you fail to start a new pill pack, you should continue on with pills for that cycle and use a backup contraceptive for 7 days
- Extensive information can be found at: www.opr.princeton.edu/ec, including background information in English and Spanish
- Check the expiration date of the package before using
- Take the first dose as soon as possible and the second dose 12 hours later
- See the following table for doses using combined oral contraceptives as emergency contraception

Dosages for combined oral contraceptives (COCs) as emergency contraception

BRAND OF COMBINED PILL	FIRST DOSE (# OF PILLS)	SECOND DOSE (# OF PILLS)
PREVEN™ or Ovral	2 pills: blue/white	2 pills: blue/white
Lo-Ovral, Nordette, Levlen, Triphasil, Trilevlen, Levora, or Trivora	4 pills Lo-Ovral: white pills Nordette: light-orange Levlen: yellow-orange Levora: pink Triphasil: yellow Trilevlen: yellow Trivora: pink	4 pills Lo-Ovral: white pills Nordette: light-orange Levlen: yellow-orange Levora: pink Triphasil: yellow Trilevlen: yellow Trivora: pink
Alesse Levlite	5 pink pills 5 pink pills	5 pills: pink 5 pills: pink

Dosages for progestin-only pills (POPs) as emergency contraception

Progestin-Only Pill	First Dose (# of pills)	Second Dose (# of pills)
PLAN B **OR** Ovrette (contains levonorgestrel)	1 tablet 20 yellow pills	1 tablet 20 yellow pills

Note: Norplant and Depo-Provera **cannot** be used as emergency contraception
See page 69 for information on using progestin-only pills as emergency contraception. Progestin-only pills (PLAN B or Ovrette) are more effective and less likely to cause nausea or vomiting than combined pills.

WHAT GUIDELINES DO I NEED TO FOLLOW?

• Nausea (50%) and vomiting (20%) are most common side effects:
  • Take an antinausea medicine such as Dramamine II or Bonine (over-the-counter) or Antivert (prescription). Take two 25-milligram tablets 1 hour before first ECP dose. This medicine decreases nausea and vomiting but causes drowsiness in about one-third of women
  • Other over-the-counter drugs decrease nausea (Marezine, Dramamine, Benadryl) but do not last 24 hours
• Swallow first dose of pills within 72 hours of unprotected intercourse (time first dose so that second dose 12 hours later is at a convenient time, such as 7 a.m. and 7 p.m.)
• Swallow second dose of pills 12 hours later
• Next period may be early, on time or late
• If your period does not come within 21 days (or is more than 1 week late), see your clinician for an exam and pregnancy test. (If it is positive, you still have the options of having an abortion, carrying pregnancy to term, keeping the baby, or adoption)
• Do not have unprotected sex after using emergency contraception
• Start routine and reliable contraception as soon as possible. Use condoms for best protection against infection

Starting Regular Use of Birth Control Pills After Their Use as Emergency Contraception:
- *One approach* is to wait until your next period and then start regular pills. In this case, your prescription for emergency contraception using Lo-Ovral might read:
  - **Rx:** *Antivert 50 milligrams: take one tablet as soon as possible*
    Lo-Ovral: Take 4 tablets 1 hour later. Then take 4 tablets 12 hours after your first dose of Lo-Ovral. Use a backup method until your next period. Start a new package of pills on the day after your period begins. Take remainder of package, one pill a day.
- *A second approach* is to start taking combined pills the day after the second dose of emergency contraception. In this case your prescription might read:
  - **Rx:** *Antivert 50 milligrams: take one tablet as soon as possible*
    Lo-Ovral: Take 4 tablets 1 hour later. Take 4 tablets 12 hours later after your first dose of Lo-Ovral. Take one pill a day starting the next morning. Use backup contraceptive for 7 days.

AFTER TAKING EMERGENCY CONTRACEPTION, ASK YOURSELF:

Following are important questions to help you evaluate your use of emergency contraception. If you answer "yes" to any question, talk to your clinician to figure out the best solution for you.

☐ Have I missed an expected period since taking emergency contraception?

☐ Do I think I may be pregnant?

☐ What contraceptive do I want to use now?

WHAT HAPPENS IF:

I vomit or am nauseated? Antinausea medicine may be taken before or after taking emergency contraception. Vomiting that is caused by emergency contraception probably means that enough of the hormones reached the bloodstream to be an effective contraceptive. (Most experts recommend another dose of pills if you vomit within 1 hour of taking first dose).

It is likely that if ECPs are placed directly in the vagina the hormone(s) will be well absorbed; this may be done if vomiting occurs in the first hour or two following a dose of emergency contraceptive pills (see page 156).

I don't get my period? If your period does not come in 21 days (or more than 7 days after the expected day for your period to begin), suspect pregnancy and get a pregnancy test.

I get pregnant in spite of using emergency contraception? If there is a pregnancy the hormones in combined pills will not cause birth defects *[IPPF, 1997]*.

WHAT IF I WANT TO GET PREGNANT AFTER USING EMERGENCY CONTRACEPTIVE PILLS?

Fertility returns after next period.

COPPER T 380-A: MOST EFFECTIVE OF THE AVAILABLE EMERGENCY OPTIONS

- Women wanting the most effective approach should consider IUD insertion. It has about one-tenth the failure rate of pills
- Prevents 99% of the pregnancies that would have occurred from this single act of intercourse. If 1000 women have unprotected intercourse in the middle 2 weeks of cycle, 80 would become pregnant **without** emergency contraception, but only 1 will become pregnant if a Copper T 380-A is inserted as emergency contraception
- May interfere with implantation or prevent fertilization
- Precautions for IUD use are same as for woman considering IUD as ongoing contraceptive (see chapter 25)
- Use of IUD may be long-term contraceptive for women, including some women who have never had a child (see chapter 25 for full information on IUDs)

- May be used by some women who cannot take pills
- Inserted into the uterus exactly as it would be for ongoing contraception
- Fertility returns immediately after IUD is removed
- If a woman has never given birth or has multiple partners, it may be wise to remove the IUD after 1-2 normal cycles and start a different long-term method because IUDs do not protect against infections that may lead to infertility

RU-486 OR MIFEPRISTONE

NOT AVAILABLE TO WOMEN IN THE US!

- Virtually 100% effective, but not currently an emergency contraception option in the USA
- Single dose of 600 milligrams within 72 hours of unprotected intercourse is extremely effective
- A recent study found that a 10 milligram dose of RU-486 may be as effective as a 600 milligram dose
- Contains antiprogestin that blocks the effects of the hormone progesterone, stops ovulation or slows the growth of the uterine lining (depending on whether it is taken before or after ovulation)
- Fertility returns after your next period
- Might delay your next period

Ask your clinician about getting emergency contraceptive pills in advance so you have them at home in case you need them.

EMERGENCY CONTRACEPTION:
Progestin-Only Pills (PLAN B or Ovrette)

You have had unprotected intercourse

↓

Within 72 hours, take your first dose of your progestin-only contraceptive:
1 tablet of PLAN B **OR** Ovrette 20 tablets
NOTE: Check expiration date on pills before you take them

↓

12 hours later repeat same dose:
1 tablet of PLAN B **OR** 20 tablets of Ovrette

↓

Use a backup contraceptive until next period

↓

Period within 21 days

↙ ↘

YES: Start and continue contraceptive of your choice—a method you will use consistently and correctly

NO: See clinician and have a pregnancy test done

NOTE: Nausea and vomiting are less likely to occur in women using progestin-only pills as emergency contraception than in women using combined pills. Anti-nausea medicine is not included in this flowchart but may be necessary if nausea or vomiting occurs after the first dose of progestin-only pills. It is probably as effective to place emergency contraceptive pills in the vagina if vomiting occurs from taking the hormones in birth control pills.

Emergency contraception using combined oral contraceptives (COCs). Ask your clinician about getting emergency contraceptive pills *in advance* so that you have them at home in case you need them.

EMERGENCY CONTRACEPTION:
Combined Oral Contraceptive Pills

Within 72 hours of unprotected or inadequately protected intercourse (as soon as possible)

↓

First, take anti-nausea medicine: (Dramamine II by prescription or Bonine over-the-counter)*

↓

One hour later, first dose of combined pills:
1) PREVEN (2 light blue pills) or Ovral (2 white pills) **OR**
2) Triphasil (yellow), Trilevlen (yellow), or Trivora (yellow), Lo-Ovral (white), Nordette (light-orange), Levlen (light-orange), or Levora (white): 4 pills **OR**
3) Alesse (pink) or Levlite (pink): 5 pills
NOTE: Check expiration date on pills before you take them

↓

12 hours later repeat same dose

↓

Use a contraceptive method until next period

↓

Menstrual period within 21 days

↙   ↘

YES: Start contraceptive of your choice— a method you will use consistently and correctly

NO: See a clinician and have pregnancy test

NOTE: If anti-nausea medicine is **NOT** taken before the first dose of emergency contraception, you can take it after the first dose, if nausea is severe or if you vomit. It is probably as effective to place emergency contraceptive pills in the vagina if vomiting occurs from taking the hormones in birth control pills.

*Meclizine hydrochloride is recommended because it lasts for 24 hours. It is available over the counter as <u>Bonine</u> and as <u>Dramamine II.</u> It is available by prescription as <u>Antivert.</u> Other medicines to prevent nausea may be prescribed (ask your clinician).

EMERGENCY CONTRACEPTION:
Copper T 380-A IUD

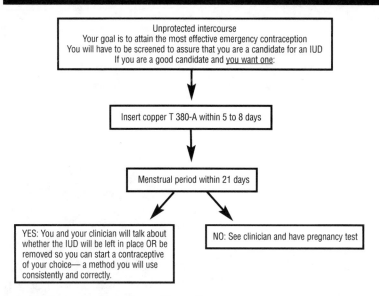

Unprotected intercourse
Your goal is to attain the most effective emergency contraception
You will have to be screened to assure that you are a candidate for an IUD
If you are a good candidate and <u>you want one</u>:

Insert copper T 380-A within 5 to 8 days

Menstrual period within 21 days

YES: You and your clinician will talk about whether the IUD will be left in place OR be removed so you can start a contraceptive of your choice— a method you will use consistently and correctly.

NO: See clinician and have pregnancy test

NOTE: The Copper T 380-A IUD may be inserted up to the time of implantation— about 5 days after ovulation— to prevent pregnancy. Thus, if you had unprotected intercourse 3 days before ovulation in that cycle, the IUD could be inserted up to 8 days after intercourse to prevent pregnancy.

If you have any questions, ask us at...
www.managingcontraception.com

What About an IUD?

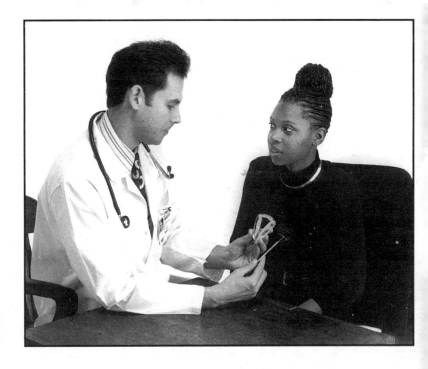

For a couple with a child or two wanting excellent contraception and not at risk for infection, an intrauterine device (IUD) is a marvelous method. While 15-25% of couples in Europe use IUDs, only 1-2% of couples in the United States use this effective, long-term and reversible method.

Talk to your clinician if you are interested in learning more or if you would like to find out if you are a candidate for an IUD.

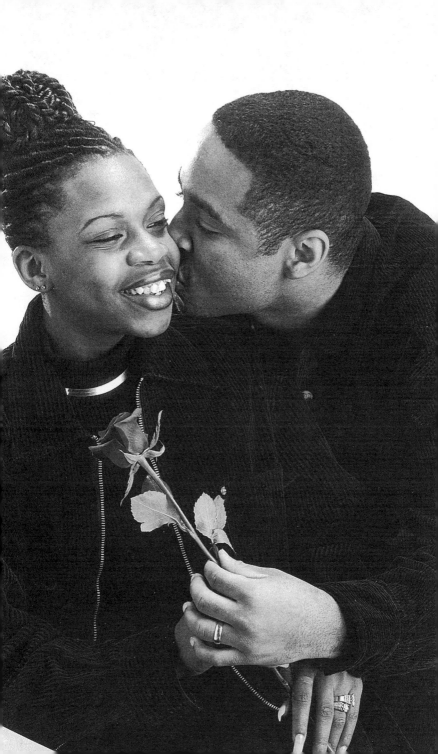

THE COPPER T 380-A IUD (Paragard)

WHAT IS THE COPPER T 380-A IUD?

It is a T-shaped IUD made of polyethylene. Each horizontal arm of the IUD has a covering of copper. Fine copper wire is wound around the vertical stem. String that is clear or whitish is knotted after passing through a hole in the stem, creating double strings that hang from lower end of the IUD.

HOW EFFECTIVE IS THE COPPER T 380-A IUD?

Perfect-use failure rate in first year: 0.6% (Of every 1000 women who used this method for one year, only 6 will become pregnant in the first year of use)

Typical-use failure rate in first year: 0.8%

• Approved for 10 years; effective for at least 12 years.
• Ectopic pregnancies *reduced* not increased
• Continuing users after 1 year: 78%

[Trussell J, Contraceptive Technology, 1998]

HOW DOES THE COPPER T 380-A IUD WORK?

Mainly this IUD causes few sperm to reach the egg. Secondly, if sperm reach the egg, the IUD reduces the ability of sperm to fertilize the egg. Thirdly, implantation is prevented should fertilization occur. **Ovulation is not affected nor does the IUD cause an abortion (disruption after implantation).**

HOW MUCH DOES THE COPPER T 380-A IUD COST?

	Managed care setting	*Public provider setting*
Device	$184	$109
Insertion	207	64.42
Removal	70	10.80

[Trussell, 1995; Smith, 1993]

NOTE: In five private offices in Atlanta, the average price of insertion was $305 in January 1999. The range was from $175 to $500 (including payment for the IUD).

WHAT ARE THE ADVANTAGES OF THE COPPER T 380-A IUD?

Menstrual
• Can be used by some women who cannot take estrogen (no hormonal side effects)
• May be inserted right after birth and at any time in a woman's cycle when it is reasonably certain she is not pregnant

Sexual/psychological:
• Nothing to do at the time of sex or on a daily basis
• Intercourse may be enjoyed more because of the decreased risk of pregnancy

Cancers, tumors, and masses:
• Decreased risk for uterine cancer found in 5 out of 6 studies of IUDs [Grimes, 1998]
• Some evidence that IUDs protect against cervical cancer

Other:
- The most effective emergency contraceptive method in the United States (1 pregnancy per 1000 insertions as emergency contraception)
- Lasts so long and is so effective that this IUD has been called "reversible sterilization"
- Offers at least 12 years of effective protection (FDA labeling states that it is effective for 10 years)
- Prevents ectopic pregnancies: 0.2 ectopic pregnancies per 1000 woman-years of use of Copper T 380-A compared to 3.0 to 4.5 ectopic pregnancies per 1000 woman-years in women not using a contraceptive method
- May be used by breastfeeding women
- Over time the cost is very low; after 2 years, it is the most cost-effective method
- Only have to check strings once a month

WHAT ARE THE DISADVANTAGES OF THE COPPER T 380-A IUD?
Menstrual
- Clinician must insert object into uterus
- Increased spotting or heavy periods
- Increased dysmenorrhea (cramping and pain during periods)
- About 12% of women get the IUD taken out because of bleeding or pain
- None of the potential *benefits* of hormonal contraceptives

Sexual/psychological
- Object must be inserted into uterus
- Some women do not like the idea of an object being inserted and remaining in the uterus
- Some men can feel the string during intercourse
- Some women do not like to put a finger into the vagina to check for string

Cancers, tumors, masses: None
Other:
- It is expensive to have an IUD inserted
- 5.7% of Copper 380-A IUDs come out of the uterus in the first year (11.3% over 5 years)
- Offers no protection against STIs; you are not a candidate if you have an infection, including HIV/AIDS, or if you are at risk of infection. If you are concerned about infection, use a condom each time you have intercourse
- You may have pain during insertion and removal; possible continued discomfort

WHAT ARE THE RISKS OF THE COPPER T 380-A IUD?
- Pelvic inflammatory disease (PID), which causes inflamed fallopian tubes. This is rare after the first 20 days (rate: 9.6/1000)
- Fainting during insertion (rare)
- Allergy to copper (rare)
- Punctured uterus during insertion (rare)
- Lost IUD strings
- If you get pregnant when an IUD is in place, have it removed right away if pregnancy is early and IUD strings are visible
  - If IUD remains in place, about 50% of pregnancies end in miscarriage
  - If IUD is removed, about 25% of pregnancies end in miscarriage
  - Risk for severe pelvic infections increases if IUD is left in place in a pregnant woman

IS THE COPPER T 380-A IUD THE RIGHT METHOD FOR ME?

Ask yourself the questions below and discuss them with your clinician. If you answer NO to ALL of the questions, then you probably CAN use an IUD if you want. If you answer YES to a question below, follow the instructions.

1. Do you think you are pregnant?

☐ No   ☐ Yes   If yes, your clinician needs to do a pregnancy test. If you are not sure, an IUD cannot be inserted. You can use condoms and/or spermicide until you are reasonably sure that you are not pregnant.

2. Have you NEVER had a child?

☐ No   ☐ Yes   If yes, other methods that offer more protection against infection and pelvic inflammatory disease (PID) may be better options in order to protect your future fertility. Return of fertility, however, is excellent for most women after IUD use. Women who have had a baby tend to tolerate an IUD better than women who have never had a baby. This is a decision that you need to make along with your health care provider.

3. In the last 3 months have you had vaginal bleeding that is unusual for you, particularly between periods or after sex?

☐ No   ☐ Yes   If yes, that may suggest a medical problem and suggests the IUD should not be inserted until the problem is diagnosed.

4. Did you have an infection following childbirth?

☐ No   ☐ Yes   If you had pelvic inflammatory disease (PID) or puerperal sepsis (genital tract infection during the first 42 days after childbirth), the IUD should not be inserted. You can choose another effective method until the infection is completely healed.

5. Have you had a sexually transmitted infection (STI) in the last 3 months? Do you have an STI, or any other infection in the female organs now? (Symptoms of pelvic inflammatory disease (PID) include pain in the lower abdomen and possibly abnormal vaginal discharge, fever, or frequent urination with burning)

☐ No   ☐ Yes   If yes, IUD cannot be inserted now. Use condoms for STI protection. You and your partner need to be treated for infection. If you are not planning another pregnancy, IUD can be inserted 3 months after cure unless it is likely that you will get another infection.

6. Have you had pelvic inflammatory disease (PID) since your last pregnancy?

☐ No   ☐ Yes   If you are still at risk for PID or STIs, you are probably not a candidate. Your clinician can help you choose another method.

7. Do you think you might get an STI in future? Do you or your partner have more than one sex partner?

☐ No   ☐ Yes   If you are at risk of STIs, they can lead to infertility. Use condoms for STI protection. Do not have an IUD inserted. Your clinician can help you choose another method.

8. Do you have any cancer in the female organs or pelvic tuberculosis?

☐ No   ☐ Yes   If you have known untreated cervical, uterine, or ovarian cancer, benign or malignant trophoblast disease or pelvic tuberculosis, is probably not advisable to use an IUD.

9. Do you think you may be infected with HIV? Do you have AIDS?

☐ No   ☐ Yes   If you have AIDS, are infected with HIV, or are being treated with any medicines that make your body less able to fight infections, it may not be advisable to use an IUD. Consider choosing another effective method. Whatever method you choose, it is important to use condoms in order to avoid passing HIV to your partner(s).

WHO CAN USE THE COPPER T 380-A IUD?

Women who:

- Want effective, safe, and intermediate-to long-term contraception
- Will use condoms if at risk of infection
- Have a reason to avoid estrogen or progestin hormones
- Need the most effective emergency contraceptive currently available
- Want an IUD after birth, miscarriage, or pregnancy termination (abortion) as long as there was no sign of infection with or after the event
- Have a past history of ectopic pregnancy (because IUD can help prevent ectopic pregnancy; although combined pills are a better option)
- Do not have an active pelvic infection, pelvic tenderness, cervical discharge with pus, or a recent proven sexually transmitted infection (but some clinicians would insert IUD if infection has been fully treated)
- Are in a mutually faithful, monogamous relationship and who have never had a baby and may want children in the future

What About Adolescents? There is some concern about future fertility because the risk of infection is high among adolescents. Other contraceptives may be a better option because they have protective effects against infection.

HOW DO I START THE METHOD?

- Most insertions are during your period or within 5 to 7 days of the start of your period
- If no risk of pregnancy, an IUD may be inserted at other times but you will need to use a back up method for the rest of your cycle
- If the IUD is inserted at a time when you do not have your period, there is a reduced risk of the uterus pushing the IUD out
- Women tend to have fewer problems leading them to get the IUD removed if it is inserted midcycle (ovulation)
- If any question of pregnancy exists, have a pregnancy test done or wait to insert the IUD until after your next period
- Taking antibiotics before insertion has shown little or no benefit in reducing the risk of infection. Each clinic develops its own policy

WHAT HAPPENS DURING INSERTION AND REMOVAL?

- Everything done at time of insertion and removal should be done slowly and gently
- Local anesthesia can help with pain if you have not given birth, have a narrow cervix, or have a history of fainting—ask your clinician
- Your clinician may use a substance called laminaria to open your cervix slightly (usually, this is not necessary)
- You should be given a part of the trimmed IUD strings and instructed on how to check for your IUD strings once it is in place. Take it home with you to remind you to check your IUD strings each month after your period
- It may be easier to remove the IUD during your period
- At the time of removal, your clinician will use a special instrument to gently pull on the strings and remove the IUD

How the IUD Is Inserted

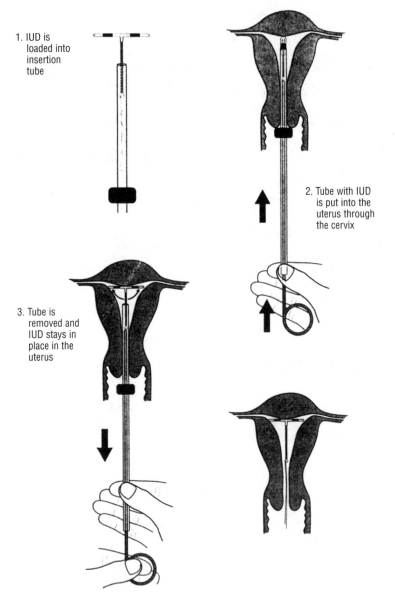

1. IUD is loaded into insertion tube

2. Tube with IUD is put into the uterus through the cervix

3. Tube is removed and IUD stays in place in the uterus

[Speroff L, Darney P. A clinical guide for contraception. 2nd ed. Baltimore: Williams & Wilkins, 1996:215.]

Copper T 380-A should be removed if:
- You want the IUD out for any reason
- You are pregnant and the strings are visible
- You have a serious infection (even after taking antibiotics)
- IUD is partially expelled (pushed out of uterus)
- You have severe pain or heavy bleeding
- You have reached menopause (1 year after last period)
- After the life span of the IUD has elapsed: Copper T 380-A is effective for at least 12 years, but is FDA-approved for 10 years
- You are being treated for cancer of the uterus or cervix
- If you have one of the following warning signs you need to be evaluated. Your IUD may need to be removed:

"Early IUD warning signs"

Caution:

P • Period late (pregnancy), abnormal spotting or bleeding
A • Abdominal pain, pain with intercourse
I • Infection exposure (any STI), abnormal discharge
N • Not feeling well, fever, chills
S • String missing, shorter or longer

WHAT GUIDELINES DO I NEED TO FOLLOW?

- If cramps or pain are a problem, take ibuprofen 200-400 milligrams, orally, every 4-8 hours at the beginning of your next 3 periods (for 3-4 days) after initial insertion
- Check for the IUD strings after each monthly period (some women check strings less often than this; frequent checks are most important in the year after insertion)
- If bleeding bothers you, contact your clinician; there are medicines that can make the bleeding better (or it may be a sign that you need to have your IUD removed)
- Consider bringing a friend or partner to drive you home after the IUD is inserted
- Return if you develop one of the warning signals (see "PAINS" above)
- Make an appointment at your clinic for the week after your next period. Your clinician can make sure the IUD has not been pushed out

DO I NEED TO CONSULT MY CLINICIAN? ASK YOURSELF:

Following are important questions to help you evaluate your use of IUDs. If you answer "yes" to any question, talk to your provider to figure out the best solution for you.

☐ Do I have questions about my IUD?
☐ Am I having any problems at all with my IUD?
☐ Have I had intercourse with a new partner since my IUD was inserted?
   If yes, with how many partners? Am I at risk of infection?
☐ Do I want to have my IUD removed?
☐ Do I want to become pregnant soon?
☐ Do I have any warning signs? (remember the word "PAINS")

WHAT HAPPENS IF:

I have spotting, bleeding, severe bleeding (hemorrhaging), or anemia (low red blood cell count)? Go for a clinical exam if bleeding is heavy or if you are concerned. Taking an iron supplement may help if your iron is low or if bleeding is heavy. During the exam, your clinician needs to make sure the IUD has not been partially pushed out, especially if you are bleeding at the time of the exam. If you have any signs of pregnancy, a test should be done. Medicines such as ibuprofen may help control the bleeding. If the bleeding lasts longer than 3 months, you need to be examined for infections or tumors, start taking an iron supplement, or try several cycles of combined pills to regulate the bleeding. You may also want to consider having the IUD removed. The IUD should be removed *if you want it taken out*, if the bleeding is related to endometriosis, or if you are over 40 years old and need to be examined for cancer of the uterus.

I have cramping and/or pain? A pain reliever (like ibuprofen) or several cycles of combined pills may decrease the discomfort. If pain during insertion is severe and continues, or if pain increases and your abdomen is tender, the IUD may have punctured your uterus. The IUD needs to be taken out if pain is caused by endometriosis, partial expulsion, perforation, related to fainting after insertion, or if you are pregnant and the IUD strings are present. If the IUD is outside of the uterus, surgery is needed.

My IUD is partially or completely pushed out? Your clinician needs to make sure you are not pregnant and that the IUD has not perforated your uterus. Ultrasound can be used to find the IUD. Another IUD can be inserted if there are no signs of infection or pregnancy. The IUD should be removed if it has been partially or completely pushed out or if you are pregnant and the IUD strings are visible.

My partner is irritated by the IUD strings? This is usually because the strings are too long. Your clinician can trim the strings (so they do not come out of the cervix) and needs to record their length and tell you. You may want to consider removing the IUD or leaving the strings longer. It may simply help to move the strings to another position. Your clinician can show you how to do this yourself.

The strings are missing or I cannot feel them? The strings are usually there, but you may need more information on how to find them. If your clinician cannot find the strings and you are not pregnant, an ultrasound is used to try to find the IUD and make sure it has not been pushed out. Use a backup contraceptive until you have been examined for this problem.

I get pregnant? If you are having a miscarriage, your clinician needs to remove the IUD and will probably give you antibiotics for 7 days and pain relievers if pain is severe. If you want an abortion and it can be performed quickly, your clinician may refer you and the IUD will be taken out at the time of the abortion. If you are considering an abortion, the IUD needs to be removed right away if the strings are present. If you want to continue the pregnancy, the IUD should be removed if strings are present. If the strings are not there, ultrasound can be used to find it. If the ultrasound demonstrates that the IUD is in the uterus, it may stay there; however, you need to be watched closely for infection and you may be at risk of preterm labor. If the IUD remains in place, about 50% of pregnancies end in miscarriage; if the IUD is removed, about 25% of pregnancies end in miscarriage.

My uterus or cervix is punctured or the IUD gets embedded? If perforation happens during insertion, your clinician needs to stop the procedure, take the IUD out, and give you another method. You will also need to be watched (probably for 2-4 hours) for internal bleeding. If you are OK after 2-4 hours, you may go home (probably with a prescribed course of oral antibiotics). You may return after 1 week to have another IUD put in (or after your next period).

I get pelvic inflammatory disease (PID)? Although some clinicians leave the IUD in place if the infection is mild, most experts say it should be taken out. In mild PID, antibiotics will nearly always be given, especially if the IUD is left in place. The IUD should not be put in again if you are at risk of sexually transmitted infections. If you have moderate to severe pelvic inflammatory disease, the IUD must be taken out. If you are pregnant and have signs of pelvic inflammatory disease, you need to take antibiotics and your clinician will probably recommend that your IUD be taken out (with your consent).

WHAT IF I WANT TO GET PREGNANT AFTER USING THE COPPER T 380-A IUD?
• Most women who stop using the Copper T-380A IUD are able to become pregnant quickly (e.g., that night if during ovulation)

PROGESTERONE IUD (PROGESTASERT SYSTEM)

WHAT IS THE PROGESTERONE IUD?
A T-shaped IUD that goes into uterus and releases 65 micrograms of progesterone per day. The "T" contains 38 milligrams of progesterone and some barium sulfate (so it can be seen on X-rays). It has blue-black double strings and is placed into the uterus using a technique different than for the Copper T 380-A. It is not effective for as long as the Copper T 380-A (approved for 1 year in the U.S. and for 18 months in France).

HOW EFFECTIVE IS THE PROGESTERONE IUD?
Perfect-use failure rate in first year: 1.5%
Typical-use failure rate in first year: 2.0%
Continuation rate at 1 year: 81% *[Trussell J, Contraceptive Technology, 1998]*
• Approved for one year of contraceptive protection (18 months in France)

HOW DOES THE PROGESTERONE IUD WORK?
It causes cervical mucus to become thicker, preventing sperm from reaching the egg. Changes in the fluid in the uterus and fallopian tubes stop sperm movement. The IUD prevents the lining of the uterus from growing to its full capacity, which makes it less likely that a fertilized egg will implant. It may also stop ovulation.

COST:

	Managed-Care Setting	*Public Provider Setting*
IUD	$82/year	$82/year
Insertion	207/year	62/year
Removal	70/year	10/year
		[Trussell, 1995; Smith, 1993]

WHAT ARE THE ADVANTAGES OF THE PROGESTERONE IUD?
Menstrual:
- May decrease blood flow during periods (on average)
- Decreases the pain some women have during periods

Sexual/psychological:
- Nothing to do on a daily basis or during sexual activity
- Sex may be enjoyed more because there is less risk of pregnancy

Cancers, tumors, and masses: None

Other:
- Safe and effective for 1 year
- May be used by some women who cannot take estrogen; no overall effects
- May protect against pelvic inflammatory disease (PID)

WHAT ARE THE DISADVANTAGES OF THE PROGESTERONE IUD?
Menstrual:
- Increases number of days some women have spotting
- Some women do not get their periods (strongly suspect pregnancy if a missed period follows consistently regular cycles. See a clinician for a pregnancy test)

Sexual/psychological: None

Cancer, tumors, and masses: None

Other:
- Offers no protection against sexually transmitted infections
- Object must be inserted into uterus every year
- May be expelled (pushed out)
- Pain during day of insertion or removal; could be painful for a few days after removal

WHAT ARE THE RISKS OF THE PROGESTERONE IUD?
- There is a slightly increased risk of pelvic inflammatory disease (PID) at the time of insertion
- Large, painful ovarian cysts (rare problem)

IS THE PROGESTERONE IUD THE RIGHT METHOD FOR ME?
Similar checklist to that of the Copper T 380-A (see page 80). Progesterone IUD is a good option for women with heavy or painful periods.

WHO CAN USE THE PROGESTERONE IUD?
Women who:
- Will use condoms if at risk for infection
- Want effective, safe, and intermediate-to long-term contraception
- Have a reason to avoid estrogen
- Have excessive or irregular bleeding from fibroids (benign tumors in the uterus) or from another known cause
- Need to take a progestin for hormone replacement therapy and cannot take other progestins (the progesterone IUD is not FDA approved for this use but it can still be used—ask your clinician)
- Do not have an active pelvic infection, pelvic tenderness, cervical discharge with pus, or a recent proven sexually transmitted infection (some clinicians would insert IUD if infection has been fully treated)
- Do not have a severely abnormal uterus, active liver disease or liver tumor, history of bacterial heart infection, any heart valve replacement, or a severe problem with the immune system

What About Adolescents? Because rates of sexually transmitted infections are high among teens, there is some concern regarding the return to fertility (if a teen gets an infection and develops pelvic inflammatory disease—PID). Other contraceptives may be a better option.

HOW DO I START THE METHOD?

- Most clinics insert the IUD during a woman's period or within 7 days of the start of the period
- If you are sure you are not pregnant, it is OK to insert an IUD at other times; backup contraceptive should be used for the rest of the cycle
- Taking antibiotics before inserting an IUD has shown little or no benefit. Each clinic develops its own policy

WHAT GUIDELINES DO I NEED TO FOLLOW?

- Check for the strings of the IUD after each monthly period
- If bleeding pattern is bothersome, contact your clinician; there are medicines that may make the pattern of bleeding better for you

DO I NEED TO CONSULT MY CLINICIAN? ASK YOURSELF:

IUD Checklist: See questions listed for Copper T 380-A users on page 83.

WHAT HAPPENS IF:

I do not get my period? Not getting your period is a normal side effect of the progesterone IUD and is not harmful. If you have signs of pregnancy, you need to have a pregnancy test done. If you are still worried about not getting a period, it may help to take a few cycles of combined pills, or you can have the IUD taken out.

I have spotting or bleeding between monthly periods? Irregular bleeding is a normal side effect of the IUD and is not harmful. If it really is a problem for you, taking a few cycles of combined pills OR a medicine such as ibuprofen may help. Your clinician needs to make sure you do not have an ectopic pregnancy or infection, including pelvic inflammatory disease (PID). If spotting or bleeding happens after you have intercourse, you should be checked for infection. The IUD should also be checked to make sure it has not been pushed out.

I have very heavy bleeding or the bleeding lasts for a long time? Your clinician needs to check to see if the IUD has been pushed out. If the bleeding is really a problem for you, taking a few cycles of combined pills OR a medicine such as ibuprofen may help. Blood testing may be necessary in some cases.

I have severe pain in my lower abdomen? You need to be treated or referred if the pain is from a pelvic infection, an ectopic pregnancy or another severe problem. If you have ovarian cysts, the IUD can stay in place because these cysts usually go away without surgery. Go back to your clinician a few days after you are checked for pain and in 3 weeks to 2 months to be sure the cysts are going away.

I have pain after the IUD is inserted? Take a pain reliever (such as ibuprofen). Go back to the clinic if pain is severe or you have bad vaginal discharge.

WHAT IF I WANT TO GET PREGNANT AFTER USING THE PROGESTERONE IUD?

Immediate and excellent return of fertility after the IUD is taken out.

LEVONORGESTREL IUD (Mirena)

WHAT IS THE LEVONORGESTREL IUD?

T-shaped IUD that comes in 2 sizes and is inserted into the uterus. It releases 20 micrograms of the hormone levonorgestrel (LNg) over 8 years. Each week the levonorgestrel IUD releases about the same amount of hormone as a woman gets when she takes one or two Ovrette pills so that the overall level of hormones in a woman's body is less with the IUD than with the pills.

HOW EFFECTIVE IS THE LEVONORGESTREL IUD?

Perfect-use failure rate in first year : 0.1% (1 of every 1,000 women with a levonorgestrel IUD will become pregnant)

Typical-use failure rate in first year: 0.1% *[Trussell J, Contraceptive Technology, 1998]*
* Most effective of all reversible contraceptives; may be left in place for at least 8 years
* Studies have now shown the IUD to be effective for 10 years

HOW DOES THE LEVONORGESTREL IUD WORK?

Levonorgestrel (a hormone) causes cervical mucus to become thicker, so sperm do not reach the egg. Changes in the fluid in the uterus and fallopian tubes also stop sperm movement. The lining of the uterus does not grow to its full capacity, which prevents a fertilized egg from implanting. This IUD may also stop ovulation.

COST: Unknown; not available in the United States (as of May 2000). Some have obtained the IUD over the internet.

WHAT ARE THE ADVANTAGES OF THE LEVONORGESTREL IUD?
Menstrual:
* Some women will stop having periods and find this to be an advantage
* Decreases blood loss during periods. On average, women have about one-quarter the blood loss as before
* Women who have anemia will improve
* Painful periods generally improve

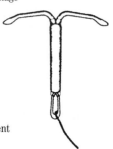

Sexual/psychological:
* There is nothing to worry about on a daily basis or during sex
* Less fear of pregnancy can make sex more pleasurable

Cancers, tumors, and masses:
* May protect against uterine cancer
* Can be used as the progestin by women on hormone replacement therapy in countries where the IUD is available

Other:
* Comes in 2 sizes (for different sized women)
* Safe, inexpensive, extremely effective (at least 8 years, but FDA labeling will say 5 years)
* Prevents ectopic pregnancies
* May decrease a woman's risk for pelvic inflammatory disease (PID) (compared to women using no method)

WHAT ARE THE DISADVANTAGES OF THE LEVONORGESTREL IUD?
Menstrual:
* Clinician must insert object into uterus
* Number of bleeding days is higher than normal for first few months (NOTE: Bleeding declines and is actually less than normal after 6 months)
* Some women will stop having periods and find this to be a disadvantage

Sexual/psychological:
- Some women feel uncomfortable checking for string
- Some women do not want an object in the uterus

Other:
- No demonstrated effectiveness as emergency contraception
- Offers no protection against infections, except perhaps the development of pelvic inflammatory disease (resulting from an untreated STI)
- IUD may be pushed out of the uterus
- The ovaries may swell because of the hormonal changes (eggs are not being regularly released). Most return to normal on their own
- Headaches, change in appetite, weight gain or loss
- Pain during or for a few days after insertion or removal

WHAT ARE THE RISKS OF THE LEVONORGESTREL IUD?
- Slight risk of pelvic inflammatory disease, but only right after insertion
- Large painful ovarian cysts can develop
- Allergy to the hormone levonorgestrel (rare)

WHO CAN USE THE LEVONORGESTREL IUD?
Women who:
- Want effective intermediate-to long-term contraception
- Will use condoms if at risk of infection
- Have no abnormal vaginal bleeding of unknown causes
- Have no current pelvic infection, pelvic tenderness, or cervical discharge with pus
- Have not had bacterial heart infection or any heart valve replacement
- Have no severe problems with the immune system
- Have excessive or irregular bleeding from fibroids (benign tumors in the uterus) (as long as the uterus is not severely distorted)
- Are going through menopause, have their uterus, are on estrogen replacement therapy, and are unable to take other progestins. These women may be able to get protection from uterine cancer from a Levonorgestrel IUD *[Raudaskoski, 1995]*

HOW DO I START THE METHOD?
- Most clinics insert IUDs during a woman's period or within 7 days of onset
- If you are not pregnant, it may be possible to insert an IUD at other times of cycle
- A local anesthetic may be required
- You need to expect menstrual cycle changes
- Take pain relievers for pain after insertion. If pain continues, you must return to the clinic
- Taking antibiotics before insertion has shown little or no clinical benefit. Each clinic develops its own policy.
- Some experts say it is acceptable for women who have had a bacterial heart infection to use the Levonorgestrel IUD as long as they take medicine to prevent another infection, but other experts (American Heart Association) say it is not unacceptable

WHAT GUIDELINES DO I NEED TO FOLLOW?
You will need to:
- Use pain relievers for 3 days of your first 3 periods
- Check for the IUD strings after each monthly period
- Return to the clinic 2-3 months after insertion for a check-up
- Contact your clinician, if your bleeding pattern is bothersome. There are medicines (pain relievers, estrogen, birth control pills) that may make the pattern of bleeding better for you

DO I NEED TO CONSULT MY CLINICIAN? ASK YOURSELF:

Following are important questions to help you evaluate your use of IUDs. If you answer "yes" to any question, talk to your clinician to figure out the best solution for you.

☐ Have my periods stopped or become irregular?
☐ Have I experienced any bleeding or spotting?
☐ Have I had heavy or prolonged bleeding?
☐ Do I have any lower abdominal pain or fever?
☐ Do I have breast pain?
☐ Have I experienced headaches, blurred vision, or dizziness?
☐ Have I been unable to feel the IUD strings?

WHAT HAPPENS IF:

I do not get my period? This is a typical and non-harmful side effect. A test for pregnancy is recommended if you have signs or symptoms of pregnancy. A cycle of low-dose combined pills may help if you are not pregnant but are still concerned after talking to your clinician.

I have spotting or bleeding between my periods? This is a typical and non-harmful side effect. Medicines such as ibuprofen may help. Your clinician needs to check for ectopic pregnancy, infection, and partial expulsion.

I have bleeding? Medicines such as ibuprofen or taking a cycle of combined pills may help. Your clinician needs to make sure the IUD is still in place.

I have abdominal pain? If due to ectopic pregnancy, you can be treated or referred. If due to ovarian cyst(s), IUD may remain in place. These cysts usually go down on their own without surgery. See your clinician again in 3 weeks (others recheck in 3 months after treatment with combined pills) to be sure that cysts are going down. If pain has other cause or cause is unknown you need to be treated or referred.

WHAT IF I WANT TO GET PREGNANT AFTER USING THE LEVONORGESTREL IUD?

Immediate and excellent return of fertility after IUD is taken out. This IUD may even have a slight protective effect against PID, which would help you in preserving fertility.

**If you have any questions,
ask us at...
www.managingcontraception.com**

WHAT ARE PROGESTIN-ONLY PILLS?

Progestin-only pills contain only a progestin and are taken daily (without hormone-free days or placebo pills). Each pill has less progestin than combined pills. Micronor and NOR-QD pills each have 0.35 milligrams of **norethindrone**, a type of progestin. Ovrette pills each have 0.075 milligrams of **norgestrel**, another type of progestin.

HOW DO PROGESTIN-ONLY PILLS WORK?

Progestin-only pills work in three ways: they stop ovulation in about 50% of cycles; they thicken cervical mucus, which stops sperm from going into the uterus; and they make the uterine lining thin, which prevents implantation.

HOW EFFECTIVE ARE PROGESTIN-ONLY PILLS?

Perfect-use failure rate in first year: 0.5% (if 200 women take POPs for 1 year, only 1 will become pregnant in the first year of use)

Typical-use failure rate in first year: 5% *[Trussell J, Contraceptive Technology, 1998]*

COST

	Managed-Care Setting	Public Provider Setting
Pills	$21.00/cycle	$17.70/cycle
Office visit	38.00	16.56

[Trussell, 1995; Smith, 1993]

WHAT ARE THE ADVANTAGES OF PROGESTIN-ONLY PILLS?

Menstrual:
- Decreased cramps and pain during periods, including problems that other treatments have not been able to help; decreased pain at the time of ovulation in some women
- Decreased blood loss during periods

Sexual/psychological:
- Possibly greater sexual enjoyment because less risk of pregnancy
- Depression may improve

Cancers, tumors, and masses:
- Possible protection against ovarian and endometrial (uterine) cancer

Other:
- Good option for breastfeeding women (right after birth or 3-6 weeks after birth), as long as milk flow has been established
- Can be used by women who cannot take pills that contain estrogen
- Can be used by women who have had thrombophlebitis (inflamed veins)
- Can be used by women who smoke and are over 35 years of age
- Easier to remember to take every single day with no days off at all
- Less nausea or vomiting than with combined pills
- Fewer headaches than experienced by women taking combined pills
- Less chloasma (facial discoloration) than combined pills
- Can be taken throughout the reproductive years and is easily reversible

WHAT ARE THE DISADVANTAGES OF PROGESTIN-ONLY PILLS?

Menstrual:
- Irregular bleeding pattern may mean more days of bleeding (but less blood loss), missed periods, very little bleeding, spotting or breakthrough bleeding
- You must take them at the same time each day. Staying on schedule is very important because progestin-only pills cause cervical mucus to thicken for only 22-24 hours.
- About 10% of women do not get periods (higher in women who are breastfeeding)

Sexual/psychological:
- In women who have depression, the depression may get worse, but is more likely to get better
- Anxiety, other mood changes, or fatigue

Cancers, tumors, and masses: May reduce risk for endometrial cancer but, overall, may have less protection against cancer than with combined pills

Other:
- No protection against vaginal infections. You must use condoms if you are at risk
- Slightly less effective than combined pills
- Expensive
- Some pharmacies may not carry progestin-only pills (but most do)
- Headaches
- Change in appetite, weight gain or loss

WHAT ARE THE RISKS OF PROGESTIN-ONLY PILLS?

- Allergy to the hormones norgestrel or norethindrone (rare)
- Breastfeeding women who have had gestational diabetes are almost 3 times as likely to develop type 2 diabetes if taking progestin-only pills than nonbreastfeeding women who are taking combined pills *[Kjos - 1998]*

ARE PROGESTIN-ONLY PILLS THE RIGHT METHOD FOR ME?

NOTE: If you have just given birth, are breastfeeding, and want to use progestin-only pills, it may be appropriate. In some places, very few women go back to the hospital or clinic after giving birth, so some clinicians will give progestin-only pills to women before they leave the hospital and have them start the pills after they get home. It is important to know, however, that there is still some disagreement among experts about starting progestin-only pills on the day you leave the hospital if you are breastfeeding. Specifically, experts disagree regarding the negative impacts immediately post-partum progestin can have on establishing breastfeeding.

Ask yourself the questions below. If you answer NO to ALL of the questions, then you CAN use progestin-only pills if you want. If you answer YES to a question below, follow the instructions; in some cases you can still use progestin-only pills.

1. Do you think you are pregnant?

☐ No   ☐ Yes   Get a pregnancy test. If you might be pregnant, use condoms or spermicide until you are reasonably sure that you are not pregnant. Then you can start progestin-only pills.

2. Do you have or have you ever had breast cancer?

☐ No   ☐ Yes   Do not take progestin-only pills. Your clinician can help you choose a method without hormones.

3. Do you have jaundice, severe liver problems or tumors?
(Are your eyes or skin unusually yellow?)

☐ No   ☐ Yes   You need to have a physical exam. If you have serious active liver disease (jaundice, painful or enlarged liver, active viral hepatitis, liver tumor), you should not take progestin-only pills and you need to be treated. Your clinician can help you choose a method without hormones.

4. Do you have vaginal bleeding that is unusual for you?

☐ No ☐ Yes If you are not likely to be pregnant, but have unexplained vaginal bleeding, you may be able to take progestin-only pills. You will need to be assessed and treated for any underlying problem as needed. Use of progestin-only pills should be reassessed after your exam or treatment.

5. Are you taking medicine for seizures? Are you taking the antibiotics rifampin or griseofulvin?

☐ No ☐ Yes If you are taking medicine for seizures or the antibiotics rifampin or griseofulvin, consistently use condoms or spermicide along with progestin-only pills because these medicines can reduce the effectiveness of the pills. If you prefer, or if you are on long-term treatment, your clinician can help you choose another effective method.

WHO CAN USE PROGESTIN-ONLY PILLS?
- Breastfeeding women who are not gestational diabetics
- Women who cannot take estrogen because they get nausea or breast tenderness, blood clots in the legs or lungs, or are smokers over age 35
- Women with migraines, particularly with focal neurological symptoms on combined pills
- Younger women and women throughout the reproductive years
- Women who will use condoms if at risk of infection
- Women who have just had an abortion
- Women who are not pregnant

SPECIAL SITUATIONS:
What if I had a previous pregnancy while using progestin-only pills correctly?
- Consider combined pills, or use a backup method at all times if you continue with this method

HOW DO I START THE METHOD?
- *If no concerns about blood clots:* you may start progestin-only pills the day you are leaving the hospital after giving birth
- *If breastfeeding:* some start progestin-only pills right after birth; others start later (see page 43)
- *After miscarriage or abortion:* start the same day
- *If having periods:* may be able to start any time you are sure you are not pregnant, however...
- *If you are not starting in the first 5 days of your period:* rule out pregnancy by getting a pregnancy test and use condoms for a week or wait until your next period
- *If switching from another method:* start progestin-only pills right away. There is no reason to wait for your period
- Use backup contraception for first 2 weeks (perhaps regularly in certain situations as above). Other women for whom a backup method should seriously be considered are women who have an ongoing risk of infection, have trouble remembering to take pills at the same time every day, and those for whom avoiding pregnancy is of the highest priority

WHAT GUIDELINES DO I NEED TO FOLLOW?

- Take one pill daily at same time each day. Start next pack the day after you finish the previous pack
- If at risk for infection, use condoms every time
- Drug and alcohol use can reduce the effectiveness of progestin-only pills. For example, being drunk or using other drugs may increase the risk of missing a pill
- If you miss a pill, use backup contraception for 7 days; consider emergency contraception depending on how eager you are to avoid unintended pregnancy

DO I NEED TO CONSULT MY CLINICIAN? ASK YOURSELF:

Following are important questions to help you evaluate your use of progestin-only pills. After starting the progestin-only pills, if you answer "yes" to any question, talk to your provider to figure out the best solution for you.

☐ Have I missed any periods? (Are there any pregnancy signs?)

☐ Have I had irregular or heavy bleeding?

☐ Have I had headaches or vision problems?

WHAT HAPPENS IF:

I do not get periods? Not getting periods while taking progestin-only pills is not harmful. You need to make sure you are not pregnant after your first missed period, especially if you have signs of pregnancy.

I have irregular bleeding? Irregular bleeding is typical and not harmful. If it bothers you, you can take medicine to help stop it (such as ibuprofen or a combined pill). You may need to be checked for ectopic pregnancy or infection. If spotting or bleeding happens after intercourse, you should be tested for infection. Call your clinician if you are concerned.

I have heavy bleeding? If cramping, pain, or bleeding bothers you, a medicine such as ibuprofen may help. These drugs decrease pain and diminish bleeding. Using a combined pill may also help. You may need to get a blood test in some cases.

I have abdominal pain? If you have an ectopic pregnancy, you need to be treated or referred. If you have ovarian cysts, you can continue progestin-only pills, knowing that these cysts usually go away on their own without surgery. Return to the clinic again in 3 weeks to be sure that the cysts are going away. If pain is due to other causes, or the cysts are causing severe problems, you need to be treated or referred.

I have severe headaches? If you have blurred vision, see flashing lights, have a temporary loss of vision, see zigzag lines, or have trouble speaking or moving clearly after starting progestin-only pills, stop taking them right away. See your clinician immediately.

WHAT HAPPENS IF I WANT TO GET PREGNANT AFTER TAKING PROGESTIN-ONLY PILLS?

There is complete and immediate return of fertility.

Taking the Road Less Traveled Sexually

Using contraceptives perfectly is not easy. It means careful attention to detail. In fact, over time, it requires incredible attention to detail. It means making contraceptive decisions thoughtfully. It means committing yourself to never taking a chance when it comes to contraception or sexually transmitted infections. Never. Here is what taking the road less traveled sexually means with regard to two specific contraceptives: pills and condoms:

PILLS: The road less traveled is to understand the effects of pills and to take pills perfectly.
- This means every day on time. If necessary, have your loved one call and remind you and check it off on HIS calendar! Make taking pills a shared responsibility.
- If pills are missed, use a back-up contraceptive until your next period. A North Carolina study found that 50% of women missed 3 or more pills in their third cycle on pills. This is a recipe for problems: spotting, breakthrough bleeding, confusion, pill discontinuation and, yes, pregnancy.
- Taken correctly, pills do much more than provide excellent contraception. Pills decrease menstrual cramps and pain, improve acne, and decrease a woman's risk of developing ovarian or endometrial cancer.
- The safety of pills improves if you watch out for and report to your clinician, the pill warning signals which can be remembered using the word "ACHES" (see page 125).

CONDOMS: For some women on pills it is important to use condoms as well. The road less traveled when it comes to condoms is to use them correctly and every time.
- Decide right now to use condoms every single time if there is any risk for the transmission of an infection.
- Negotiate this commitment to using condoms every single time in advance. You must both be committed to this course of action.
- The contract between the two of you might be: "We will never have intercourse without a condom. No exceptions." Sometimes this will mean stopping sexual intimacy in order to go get a condom.

The road less traveled sexually means commitment in advance to never taking a chance. Half of all pregnancies in the United States are unintended. Attention to details such as those noted above could dramatically reduce unintended pregnancies, abortions and infections in the new millennium. Good luck!

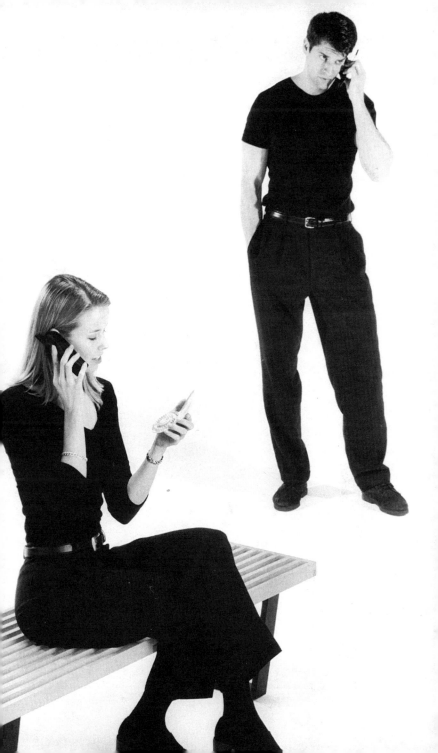

Pills: Combined Oral Contraceptives (COCs)
www.managingcontraception.com

WHAT ARE COMBINED PILLS?

These are the most commonly used birth control pills by women in
the U.S. today. Each pill has an **estrogen** and a **progestin. Ethinyl
estradiol** is the estrogen used in all pills with less than 50 micrograms; two 50-microgram pills (prescribed rarely) use the estrogen

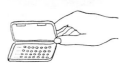

mestranol. Many different progestins are found in different pills. All pills except for one have
21 hormonally active pills followed by 7 hormone free pills (or 7 placebo pills). The exception
is Mircette which has only a 2-day hormone-free interval (after 21 days of hormones, there are
2 days of no hormones followed by 5 days of 10 micrograms of estrogen daily).

HOW EFFECTIVE ARE COMBINED PILLS?

Perfect-use failure rate in first year: 0.1% (Of every 1,000 women who take pills for 1
year, 1 will become pregnant in the first year of use)
Typical-use failure rate in first year: 5% *[Trussell J, Contraceptive Technology, 1998]*
• No backup method necessary during the hormone-free days
• Women may be able to use pills more effectively and consistently by removing or
  decreasing the pill-free period (talk to your clinician about doing this)

HOW DO COMBINED PILLS WORK?

They stop ovulation (90% to 95% of time). They also cause cervical mucus to get thicker, which
blocks sperm from getting into the uterus. The lining of the uterus does not grow to its full
capacity, which prevents implantation (embedding of fertilized egg in the lining of the uterus).

COST

	Managed Care Setting	*Public Provider Setting*
Pills	$21/pack	$17.70/pack (much lower in some clinics)
Office visit	38	16.56 (lower in many clinics)
		[Trussell, 1995; Smith, 1993]

• Costs differ from place to place, and pills with more estrogen cost more

WHAT ARE THE ADVANTAGES OF COMBINED PILLS?
Menstrual:
  • Decreased cramps and pain during periods; often more effective than other medicines
    used to treat painful periods
  • Decreased pain during ovulation
  • Decreased blood loss during periods (60% or more decrease)
  • Estrogen keeps the lining of the uterus in place so women on pills have less spotting
    than women not on pills
  • Pills are a treatment for irregular periods, heavy bleeding, and abnormal bleeding
  • Can prevent excessive bleeding in women who have a severe bleeding problem
  • You can change the cycle so you do not get your period on vacations, during exams, or on
    your honeymoon (only works with pills that use the same amount and type of hormones
    throughout the cycle)
  • You can decrease the number of cycles over time (take 3 series of 21 active pills followed
    by pill-free interval of 4 days). Doing this can decrease PMS, depression, symptoms of
    inflamed uterine lining, cyclic breast tenderness, or migraine headaches (see box on
    taking 3 or more cycles of pills without placebo pills, page 105)

Sexual/psychological:
- May enhance sexual enjoyment because less risk of pregnancy
- May make sex more spontaneous
- Depression is likely to improve or remain the same
- Interest in sex or ability to have orgasms likely to increase or remain the same

Cancers, tumors, and masses:
- *In general:* Women who are taking combined pills are less likely to get reproductive cancer in their lifetime than women who are not taking combined pills. Combined pills can protect against ovarian cancer, endometrial cancer, ovarian cysts, ectopic pregnancy, pelvic inflammatory disease (PID), anemia, and benign breast disease *[Peipert, 1993]*.
- *Breast cancer:* Most recent research shows that young women who have not given birth and are taking combined pills are slightly more likely than those who are not taking the pill to be *diagnosed* with breast cancer—about 1 in 1000 women under the age of 45. This may be because pills promote the growth of existing cancer or because women who use pills are more likely to get an exam and then be diagnosed. Breast cancers diagnosed while taking pills and in the years after a woman stops taking pills are less likely to spread to other parts of the body. Women who have taken pills and are more than 45 years old, are at NO increased risk for having breast cancer diagnosed
- *Ovarian cancer:* Women who have been taking combined pills for 4 years are 30% less likely to get ovarian cancer than women who are not taking combined pills. The longer a woman takes pills, the more protection she has against ovarian cancer. Protection lasts for years after a woman stops taking combined pills. Pills protect against ovarian cancer in women who carry the genes predisposing them to developing breast cancer to about the same extent as they do in women who do not carry these genes *[Narod, 1998]*
- *Endometrial (uterine) cancer:* Women who have been taking combined pills for at least 2 years are 40% less likely to get endometrial cancer than women who are not taking pills. The longer a woman takes pills, the more protection she has against endometrial cancer. Protection appears to continue after a woman stops taking pills
- *Colorectal cancer:* Women who are currently using combined pills and women who have used combined pills within the past 10 years are less likely than women not taking combined pills to die from colorectal cancer

Other:
- Combined pills are highly effective, available, easy to use, and reversible
- Prevent ectopic pregnancies
- Severity of pelvic inflammatory disease (PID) decreased
- May improve acne, reduce hair growth on face, and improve symptoms from cysts on the ovaries
- May or may not reduce osteoporosis and arthritis (studies have shown conflicting results)
- Can help improve endometriosis
- Probably improves bone density in women
- No harmful effects on a fetus if taken during a pregnancy by accident

WHAT ARE THE DISADVANTAGES OF COMBINED PILLS?
Menstrual:
- Spotting, mostly during the first few cycles
- More spotting in women who smoke
- Missed periods or very little bleeding with periods
- You may not get your period for 1-3 months after stopping pills (rare)

Sexual/psychological:
- May lead to depression, anxiety, fatigue, or mood changes
- Decreased sex drive or orgasm problems

Cancers, tumors, and masses:
- *Cervical cancer:* Risk of one type of cervical cancer (adenocarcinoma) increases slightly in women using combined pills. It is unclear if the risk for cervical cancer is increased by taking pills or by other factors such as having sex at a young age, having a high number of sexual partners, smoking, or if having an infection is causing a slightly higher number of cancer to be diagnosed in pill users
- *Liver tumors:* Risk increases slightly but only in those using 50 micrograms or more of estrogen. The vast majority of women (99%) in the U.S. are using less than 50 micrograms and have no increased risk of cervical cancer

Other:
- No protection against sexually transmitted infections, including HIV/AIDS. **Use condoms if at risk**
- Nausea or vomiting is possible, mostly during the first few cycles
- Increased breast size (may be advantage or disadvantage) and/or increased breast tenderness
- Increased appetite, but weight gain *due to the pill* is not common (weight loss is almost as common)
- Headaches
- High blood pressure occurs in less than 1 in 200 women
- Pill-related fluid retention may cause changes in vision that affect the fit of contact lenses (the fit can usually be adjusted by your provider)
- Depending on the office or clinic, the cost of pills may be high

WHAT ARE THE RISKS OF COMBINED PILLS?

Some women may develop deep vein thrombosis (blood clots) if they take combined pills. Although the risk of serious problems is small (1 death out of 1 million women taking combined pills each year), you need to tell your clinician before you start pills if you have had blood clots in the past, or if someone in your family has had these problems (NOTE: there is probably <u>NOT</u> an increased risk of blood clots among women using the new progestin pills containing the hormones desogestrel, gestodene or norgestimate in comparison with other combined pills). All combined pills raise triglycerides, which are building blocks for cholesterol and which can cause some increased risk of pancreatitis or heart disease.

WHO CAN USE COMBINED PILLS?

Women who:
- Can remember to take a pill every day and who can afford to buy them
- Hope to gain other advantages of pills, plus excellent contraception (women with endometriosis, severely painful periods, anemia or with strong family history of ovarian cancer)
- Range in age from just getting their periods (or rarely: for sexually active teens, even before periods begin) to menopause
- Are overweight or underweight, diabetics without vascular disease, have family history of breast cancer, are age 35 or older and non-smokers; or are smokers under age 35. Most women in these groups CAN use combined pills, but some clinicians will not give them pills

What About Adolescents?
- Combined pills may be used in sexually active adolescents even before their periods begin
- Excellent for treating teens with dysmenorrhea (painful periods are the number one reason for missing school/work)
- Pills may help acne and generally do not cause weight gain
- May benefit PMS, endometriosis and women with low estrogen levels caused by eating disorders or excessive exercise
- May cause a slight reduction in bone growth: studies have shown a 1.5% increase in bone mass in teens on combined pills versus 2.9% in teens not on pills *[Cromer, 1996]*. However, seven of 10 studies show increased bone density in women taking combined pills compared to women not taking pills

- May be used by teens who smoke, but every individual who smokes needs to be encouraged to stop smoking
- Teens need to use condoms along with pills for protection against infections
- Failure rate among teens is higher than among all other age groups (e.g., they are more likely to forget to take pills, or stop taking pills)
- It may help teens to figure out where to keep pills and how to remember to take them at the same time each day (while putting on or taking off jewelry, putting on acne medicine, or brushing teeth)

ARE COMBINED PILLS THE RIGHT METHOD FOR ME?

Ask yourself the questions below. If you answer NO to ALL of the questions, then you can use low-dose combined pills if you want. If you answer YES to a question below, follow the instructions.

1. Do you smoke cigarettes and are you age 35 or older?

☐ No   ☐ Yes   If yes, you need to stop smoking completely. If you are 35 or older and cannot or will not stop smoking (including smoking less than 15 cigarettes per day), you cannot use combined pills. Your clinician can help you choose another method without estrogen.

2. Do you have high blood pressure?

☐ No   ☐ Yes   *If your blood pressure is below 140/90*, it is probably OK for you to take combined pills. *If your blood pressure is between 140-159/90-99*, it is probably OK to take combined pills but you need to have your blood pressure checked within 1-2 months. One blood pressure reading in this range is not enough to diagnose high blood pressure. At the next reading, if it is below 140/90, it is OK to take combined pills. If it stays in the range of 140-159/90-99, combined pills are probably not the best method. But, if you choose to keep using combined pills, your blood pressure should be taken at each regular visit. *If your blood pressure is 160/100 or higher*, you cannot take combined pills. Your clinician can help you choose another method without estrogen. (Some clinicians will give combined pills if high blood pressure is under treatment and well controlled.)

3. Are you breastfeeding a baby less than 6 months old? (See page 104)

☐ No   ☐ Yes   Most experts agree that it is OK to get the combined pills you will start using when you stop nursing. (Also, get backup contraception to use while you are nursing your baby.) There is some disagreement among experts about getting combined pills and starting them when you begin to give your baby food from other sources (bottle milk or solid foods). There is a lot of disagreement among experts about starting combined pills 3-6 weeks after giving birth. The Planned Parenthood Federation of America suggests that pills can be used but that women who are nursing should wait 6 weeks to start.

4. Do you have, or have you ever had, serious problems with your heart or blood vessels, including heart attack or heart disease from blocked arteries, stroke, blood clots, severe chest pain with unusual shortness of breath, diabetes for more than 20 years, or damage to your vision, kidneys, or nervous system caused by diabetes?

☐ No   ☐ Yes   If yes, you should not take combined pills. Your clinician can help you choose another method without estrogen.

5. Do you have, or have you ever had, breast cancer?

☐ No   ☐ Yes   If yes, it is generally not recommended that you take combined pills. Your clinician can help you choose another method without hormones.

6. Do you often get bad headaches with blurred vision?

☐ No   ☐ Yes   If you get migraine headaches and have blurred vision, temporary loss of vision, see flashing lights or zigzag lines, or have trouble speaking or moving, do not take combined pills. Your clinician can help you choose another method without estrogen.

7. Are you taking medicine for seizures? Are you taking the antibiotics rifampin or griseofulvin?

☐ No   ☐ Yes   Some medicines reduce the effectiveness of the combined pills. If you are taking medicine for seizures or the antibiotics rifampin or griseofulvin, you need to use condoms or spermicide along with combined pills, or take a higher dose of combined pills (50 micrograms), or if you prefer, choose another effective method if you are on long-term treatment with these drugs.

8. Do you think you are pregnant?

☐ No   ☐ Yes   If yes, you need to take a pregnancy test. If you might be pregnant, you can use condoms or spermicide until you are reasonably certain that you are not pregnant. Then you can start combined pills. If you had unprotected sex in the past 3 days, consider emergency contraception if you are not pregnant.

9. Do you have vaginal bleeding that is unusual for you?

☐ No   ☐ Yes   If you are not likely to be pregnant but have unexplained vaginal bleeding that might be from another medical condition, you can take combined pills. Your clinician can assess and treat the condition, or refer you to someone who can do so. Your use of combined pills should be reassessed based on the cause of your vaginal bleeding.

10. Do you have jaundice, cirrhosis of the liver, or liver infection or tumor? (Are your eyes or skin unusually yellow?)

☐ No   ☐ Yes   If you have a serious liver disease, you cannot take combined pills. You need to be treated for the liver problem and your clinician can help you choose another method without hormones.

11. Do you have gallbladder disease? Have you ever had jaundice while taking combined pills (yellowish eyes or skin)?

☐ No   ☐ Yes   If you have gallbladder disease now or take medicine for gallbladder disease, or if you have had jaundice while using combined pills, you cannot take combined pills.

12. Are you planning surgery that will keep you from walking for a week or more? Have you had a baby in the past 21 days?

☐ No   ☐ Yes   Your provider can help you choose a method without estrogen (to reduce the risk of a blood clot occurring in the legs). If you are planning surgery or have just had a baby, you can get combined pills and start them later, following your clinician's instructions.

HOW DO I BEGIN TAKING OR CONTINUE USING PILLS?

- If you can take estrogen, you can take any pill below 50 micrograms
- If you are currently on a 50-microgram pill and have not tried a lower dose pill, it is a good idea to talk to your clinician about switching to a lower dose pill (If you are taking a pill with more than 35-micrograms of estrogen, there should be a clear medical reason)
- Because triphasic pills may cause confusion, the authors prefer using monophasic pills. Monophasic pills provide the same amount of estrogen and progestin in each hormonally active pill
- Combined pills are available over the counter in many countries (not in the USA)
- The following page lists a number of ways of starting pills

Starting Combined Pills in Different Situations*

BEFORE STARTING I:	WHEN DO I START?
Have no special situation; just starting or restarting combined pills	1) First day of your next period OR 2) On Sunday (which may be the day your period starts, or the Sunday after your period starts) (use backup method for 1 week) OR 3) On the day of your office visit, if you are not pregnant, you can start with appropriate pill for your time in the cycle (use backup method for 1 week)
Am having my period (see Timing Table, page 33)	1) First day of your period OR 2) On Sunday after your next period starts unless your period starts on a Sunday (in that case, start the day bleeding starts) OR 3) On the day of your office visit, if you are not pregnant you can start with appropriate pill for your time in the cycle
Have not been getting my period and am sure I am not pregnant	You can start on the day of office visit, or any day after that
Have given birth and am breastfeeding	Planned Parenthood suggests that pills can be used but that women who are nursing should wait 6 weeks to start (see page 100)
Have given birth and am not breastfeeding (after pregnancy of 24 or more weeks)	1) Day 21 after birth, OR 2) The Sunday after 21 days after birth because of increased risk for blood clots after birth
Am done with breastfeeding, but still have not had a period	1) If you gave birth less than 6 months ago, you can start pills right away or on the next Sunday. 2) If it has been more than 6 months after birth and you are not pregnant, then start pills and use a backup method for 1 week
Have had an induced, first-trimester abortion OR have had a second-trimester abortion at less than 24 weeks	Start pills on the same day (right away), the next day or the following Sunday
Want to switch from a higher dose to a lower dose combined pill	You can switch on the same day. Use a backup method for 1 week if there is a 7-day pill-free interval before taking the first lower dose combined pill
Have been taking progestin-only pills and am having periods	1) You can start on the first day of your period OR 2) On the following Sunday
Have been using Norplant implants or IUD	You can start on the day of removal or on the following Sunday
Have been using Depo-Provera (see page 33)	You can start on the last day the shot was effective (day 91) or earlier
Have been taking progestin-only pills and not getting my period	1) You can start on the day of office visit (any day) after confirming you are not pregnant OR 2) The day after you finish your progestin-only pill pack
Am having my first period after taking emergency contraception	You can start on day 1 or 2 of your period (if you are sure the flow is normal) or the day after the 2nd dose of emergency contraceptive pills

*Adapted from Guillebaud J. Contraception Today. 3rd ed. London: Martin Dunitz Ltd., 1997.

CHOOSING A PILL

(Discuss each step with your clinician)

YOU WANT TO USE "THE PILL." DO YOU:

- Smoke and are you age 35 or older?
- Have hypertension?
- Have unexplained abnormal vaginal bleeding?
- Have diabetes with known vascular complications or have you had diabetes for more than 20 years?
- Have a history of blood clots in the legs or lungs or current or past history of ischemic heart disease (except if anticoagulated)?
- Get headaches with visual or neurological symptoms or have you had a stroke?

- Have or have you had breast cancer (exceptions may be made if no evidence of disease in past 5 years)?
- Have active viral hepatitis or moderate to severe cirrhosis of the liver?
- Breastfeed fully at the present time?
- Have a history of surgery where you were immobilized within the past month?
- Have a history of gall bladder attacks while taking combined pills?
- Have a family history of thrombosis (blood clots)?

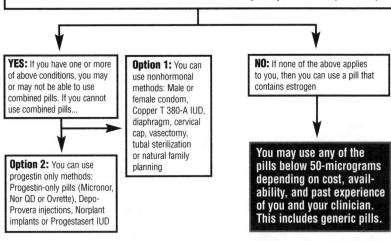

YES: If you have one or more of above conditions, you may or may not be able to use combined pills. If you cannot use combined pills...

Option 1: You can use nonhormonal methods: Male or female condom, Copper T 380-A IUD, diaphragm, cervical cap, vasectomy, tubal sterilization or natural family planning

NO: If none of the above applies to you, then you can use a pill that contains estrogen

Option 2: You can use progestin only methods: Progestin-only pills (Micronor, Nor QD or Ovrette), Depo-Provera injections, Norplant implants or Progestasert IUD

You may use any of the pills below 50-micrograms depending on cost, availability, and past experience of you and your clinician. This includes generic pills.

OTHER INFORMATION TO HELP YOU CHOOSE:

- The World Health Organization and the Food and Drug Administration both recommend using the lowest dose pill that is effective. All combined pills with less than 50 micrograms of estrogen *are* effective and safe

- Although there are no studies that show a decreased risk for deep vein thrombosis (severe blood clots in the legs) in women on 20-microgram pills, data on higher dose pills show that there is less risk of blood clots if the amount of estrogen is lower

- A 20-microgram pill may cause less nausea or breast-tenderness

- **Pill labels in Canada for all combined pills state that pills may reduce acne.** All combined pills can help improve acne. In some studies pills with the estrogens norgestimate and desogestrel were more effective in treating acne than other pills. In America only the label for Tri-Cyclen states that it can be used to treat acne

- Women need to be aware that spotting and breakthrough bleeding gets better over time. Using a different pill or brand of pill may also help if it does not get better with time (see Page 109)

- For some women, the effect of combined pills on cholesterol is a concern. Although no studies have shown that some pills work better than others in lowering cholesterol, some providers may give you a pill that contains the hormones norgestimate or desogestrel. Modicon, Brevicon, and Ovcon 35 also lead to favorable effects on lipids. Estrogen has a positive effect on the walls of blood vessels. All combined pills raise a building block of cholesterol called triglycerides

I have heard about women taking many active pills (63 monophasic pills or more) in a row with no break. What are the reasons for this?

- Migraine headaches without visual problems, ("menstrual migraine") and other problems that happen regularly during the week off hormones when you bleed
- Very heavy or painful bleeding during the week off hormones
- Severe PMS including depression
- Taking medicines which make pills less effective (anti-seizure medicines and certain antibiotics)
- Whenever you have a reason to think pills might be less effective (missing several pills a month or pregnancy even after taking pills correctly)
- If you choose to for your convenience (e.g., you want to avoid bleeding during vacation)
- Reduce pain associated with endometriosis

(Adapted from Guillebaud J. Contraception Today. 3rd ed. London: Martin Dunitz Ltd., 1997.)

WHAT IF I WANT TO TAKE COMBINED PILLS AND:

I am 35-50 years old and do not smoke? Taking combined pills may help relieve the symptoms that may come in the years before menopause (irregular, heavy, or painful periods, hot flashes, mood changes, thinning lining of the vagina). Pills with 20-micrograms of estrogen (Alesse, Levlite, LoEstrin 1/20, or Mircette) may be preferable to decrease risk of blood clotting problems.

I have ovarian cysts that keep coming back? Pills with 35 or more micrograms of estrogen might make the cysts worse than a lower dose pill. You may also change to a pill with more progestin in it or use a monophasic pill (a pill with the same amount and combination of hormones throughout the cycle). Finally consider with your clinician taking pills without a hormone-free period.

I have endometriosis? The goals in treatment are to minimize the buildup of the lining of uterus, to decrease cramping and pain during periods, to decrease back-flow of blood into the uterus, and to avoid bleeding during hormone-free periods. You might take 3 or more cycles of 21 active pills in a row (called "tricycling", see box above).

I have a family history of breast cancer? This issue is complicated, but in a review of all the studies on breast cancer and pills; no additional statistically significant risk was found for breast cancer directly related to using combined pills. Women who have the genes for breast cancer may be able to use hormonal contraceptives. You need to carefully go over the recommended schedule for mammography with your clinician and do regular breast self exams. Most organizations recommend that you have mammography performed each year after the age of 40 if you have a family history of breast cancer. Any breast masses found need to be reported to your clinician and treated or monitored. The decision is up to you. If you do want to use combined pills, a low-dose pill is best.

I am taking a medicine that affects the liver?
There are three options for a woman taking medicines that cause the liver to break down the hormone in the pill more quickly, making them less effective:
1. Take a pill that has high levels of estrogen and progestin.
2. Take 3-4 consecutive cycles of 21 active pills, followed by a shortened pill-free interval of 2-4 days. Continue this pattern.
3. Take a low dose (but not a very low dose) pill and use a backup contraceptive like condoms because the medicine can make the pills less effective.

I am taking a broad-spectrum antibiotic like tetracycline, ampicillin, or erythromycin?
There is no evidence that short or long-term use of broad-spectrum antibiotics decreases the effectiveness of low-dose combined pills in women who take them correctly. In first 2 weeks of use of these antibiotics, some providers tell women to use a backup contraceptive like condoms. Broad-spectrum antibiotics do cause estrogen levels to fall. Even though studies do not show a decrease in effectiveness, because the hormone progestin continues to work as a contraceptive, some clinicians feel that it may be wise to offer women the option of using a backup method as long as she is taking antibiotics. Illnesses that require you to take antibiotics may interfere with your body's capacity to absorb and use the pill effectively. For example, if you are vomiting, your body is less likely to absorb all the hormones in the pill. Therefore, it may be a good idea to use a backup method when you have been ill. If you are taking antibiotics for a sexually transmitted infection, it is definitely a good idea to use condoms.

I am breastfeeding? It is probably better to use progestin-only pills. If combined pills are used the authors believe it is best to use the lowest estrogen pill and to start only after breastfeeding is well established or after 6 months. It is a good idea to start combined pills or another effective contraceptive as soon as a woman starts to give her baby other food or when she starts weaning her baby from breast milk (see chapter 15, page 39).

I have high total cholesterol (close to 300)? Stop smoking if you smoke. You need to have your lipid profile measured (HDL, LDL, and triglycerides). It is possible that you may be able to start pills. If you have a low HDL/LDL ratio, choose a pill which improves the ratio (Ortho-Cyclen; Ortho Tri-cyclen; Desogen; Ortho-Cept; Ovcon 35; Mircette; Modicon or Brevicon). If you have high triglycerides (350 - 400 or greater) consider a progestin-only method. Talk to your clinician or a nutritionist about your diet and get follow-up testing of your cholesterol level.

WHAT GUIDELINES DO I NEED TO FOLLOW?
- You will need to have regular checkups once you start taking combined pills and return to your clinician to discuss any of the above problems, if you get one of the warning signs (**A**bdominal pain, **C**hest pain, **H**eadaches, **E**ye problems like blurred vision or loss of vision and **S**evere leg pain—see page 94 and page 107) or have any questions
- Take one pill at the same time each day; taking pills when you brush your teeth or doing some other regular activity can help you remember to take them; you may want to use a backup method for the first week
- Nausea and spotting (slight bleeding) are most common in the first few months of pill use
- In certain cases, some clinics will mail you your pill refills—ask your clinician
- Drugs or alcohol use can reduce the effectiveness of pills. For example, being drunk or using other drugs may increase the risk of missing a pill

DO I NEED TO CONSULT MY CLINICIAN? ASK YOURSELF:

Following are important questions to help you evaluate your use of combined pills. After starting combined pills, if you answer "yes" to any question, talk to your clinician to figure out the best solution for you.

☐ Have I had nausea or vomiting?
☐ Am I spotting or having irregular vaginal bleeding? (see page 109)
☐ Have I missed periods occasionally (no bleeding)? (see page 110)
☐ Are my breasts tender or have I found any lumps in my breasts?
☐ Have I been depressed or have I had severe anxiety or mood changes?
☐ Have I noticed a decreased interest in sex?
☐ Has my ability to have orgasms decreased?
☐ Have I gained 5 pounds or more?
☐ Has my blood pressure gone up?
☐ Have I started to smoke or increased my smoking?
☐ Am I taking medicines for seizures?
☐ Do I forget to take pills quite often? (see page 111 and 112)
☐ Have I changed sexual partners?
☐ Have I had any of the following symptoms:

ACHES: A way to remember pill danger signals (also see page 125)

Abdominal pain? Yellow skin or eyes?
Chest pain?
Headaches that are severe? (see page 113)
Eye problems: blurred vision or loss of vision?
Severe leg pain or swelling (in the calf or thigh)?

WHAT HAPPENS IF:

I have nausea? Nausea usually goes away after the first few cycles of pills. Taking pills at bedtime, with evening meal, or in the middle of a light breakfast may help. If you vomit within 1 hour of taking a pill, take an extra pill from another package. If nausea persists, switch to a 20-microgram pill (Alesse, Levlite, LoEstrin 1/20, or Mircette). If this doesn't stop the nausea, switch to a progestin-only pill.

I have spotting and/or breakthrough bleeding? (page 109) Spotting and breakthrough bleeding tend to go away after first few cycles of pills. Taking pills at the same time each day may help. Your clinician may also increase the dose of the progestin or the estrogen. Raising the estrogen step by step (Estrostep) may help or you can switch to a 30-35 microgram pill. See flow chart on page 109.

I missed one pill? (page 111) Take the forgotten pill as soon as you remember. Take next pill on schedule as you normally would. You may want to use emergency contraception or backup contraception if you absolutely do not want to get pregnant.

I miss 2 pills? See flow chart on page 112.

I miss a period while on combined pills? See flow chart on page 110.

I have headaches while on combined pills? See flow chart on page 113.

I got pregnant before while using pills correctly? Take 3 or 4 cycles of 21 active pills in a row followed by a shortened pill-free interval of 4 days. Repeat this regimen OR take 50-microgram ethinyl estradiol pill (high progestin/high estrogen pill) OR take low-dose pill, but decrease the pill-free interval to 2-4 days, and use a backup contraceptive such as condoms.

I have hot flashes in the hormone-free week? A low dose of estrogen during the hormone-free week may minimize symptoms. Take Mircette, which has only 2 estrogen-free days (although it has not been proven that this will work for hot flashes). Talk with your clinician about the possibility of taking pills without any pill-free interval.

I want to switch from combined pills to hormone replacement therapy?
See flow chart on page 114.

WHAT IF I WANT TO GET PREGNANT AFTER USING COMBINED PILLS?
- Excellent return of fertility; even if you do not ovulate or get periods for several months
- No harmful effects on a fetus if taken during a pregnancy by accident
- If you had painful, infrequent or irregular periods before using pills, this pattern may come back after stopping pills

---

**If you have any questions,
ask us at...
www.managingcontraception.com**

WHAT IF I HAVE SPOTTING/BREAKTHROUGH BLEEDING and I am taking combined pills?

You have SPOTTING or BREAKTHROUGH BLEEDING and are on combined pills.
Call or return to your clinician to find out what is going on. You will be asked/tested for the following:

Are you having pelvic pain, pain during periods, or pain during sexual intercourse?
Do you have cervicitis, pelvic inflammatory disease, cervical cancer, endometrial cancer or any other pelvic problem? Have you started any new medicines (e.g., antiseizure medicines, rifampin or griseofulvin)?

YES

NO

Other causes of spotting and/or breakthrough bleeding need to be evaluated carefully (particularly important if breakthrough bleeding or spotting happens after you have intercourse, comes with an abnormal discharge, or is painful)

Have you missed pills?

YES

NO

You may keep taking pills but need to try to stay on schedule; try to find second person to help you remember and a time of day at which you can remember to take pill every day

You may keep taking pills. Spotting may get better over time with no changes. Starting your next pack of pills on the first day of your next menstrual period may help. Changing the pill brand may help. If breakthrough bleeding is before periods, consider triphasic pill (Triphasil, Trilevlen, Tricyclen or Estrostep). If breakthrough bleeding comes after periods, consider Mircette or increase estrogen or decrease progestin. If breakthrough bleeding occurs midcycle, increase both estrogen and progestin. There is no research proving that any pill is clearly better than any other pill in stopping breakthrough bleeding. Always talk to your clinician before making any changes.

Has the bleeding gotten better or stopped completely?

YES

NO

If bleeding was stopped by taking a higher dose pill, you may be able to switch back to a lower dose pill in a few months

Consider stopping pill and choose another method if bleeding is too much of a problem

WHAT IF I HAVE MISSED ONE PERIOD
and I am taking combined pills?

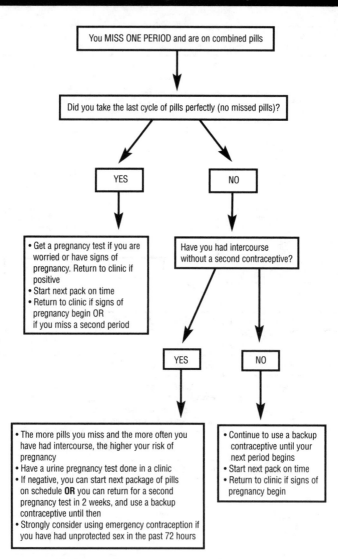

You MISS ONE PERIOD and are on combined pills

↓

Did you take the last cycle of pills perfectly (no missed pills)?

YES

- Get a pregnancy test if you are worried or have signs of pregnancy. Return to clinic if positive
- Start next pack on time
- Return to clinic if signs of pregnancy begin OR if you miss a second period

NO

Have you had intercourse without a second contraceptive?

YES

- The more pills you miss and the more often you have had intercourse, the higher your risk of pregnancy
- Have a urine pregnancy test done in a clinic
- If negative, you can start next package of pills on schedule **OR** you can return for a second pregnancy test in 2 weeks, and use a backup contraceptive until then
- Strongly consider using emergency contraception if you have had unprotected sex in the past 72 hours

NO

- Continue to use a backup contraceptive until your next period begins
- Start next pack on time
- Return to clinic if signs of pregnancy begin

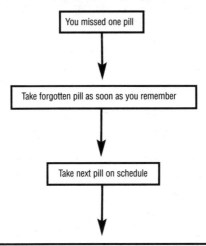

You missed one pill

Take forgotten pill as soon as you remember

Take next pill on schedule

NOTE: You can use emergency contraception OR backup contraceptives for the week following even one missed pill **if you want to do everything you can to minimize your risk for an unintended pregnancy. Call 1-888-NOT-2-LATE to learn about emergency contraceptive options and to find the phone numbers of 5 clinicians nearest to you who will prescribe emergency contraceptives.**

WHAT IF I MISS TWO PILLS?

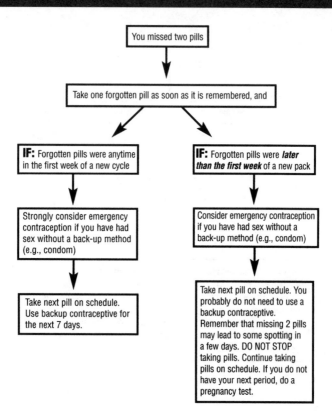

NOTE: You can use emergency contraception pills OR backup contraceptives for the week following missed pills **if you want to do everything you can to minimize your risk for an unintended pregnancy. Call 1-888-NOT-2-LATE to learn about emergency contraceptive options and to find the phone numbers of 5 clinicians nearest to you who will prescribe emergency contraceptives.**

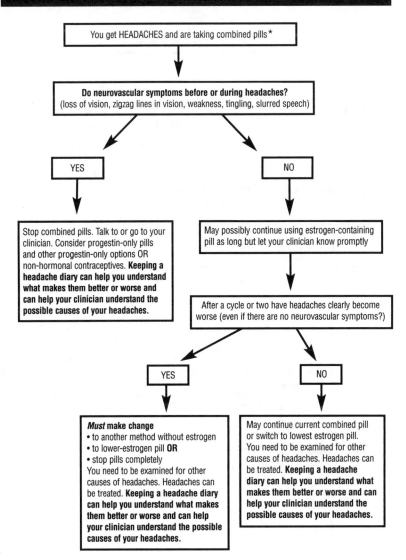

WHAT IF I GET HEADACHES
and am taking combined pills?

You get HEADACHES and are taking combined pills*

Do neurovascular symptoms before or during headaches?
(loss of vision, zigzag lines in vision, weakness, tingling, slurred speech)

YES

NO

Stop combined pills. Talk to or go to your clinician. Consider progestin-only pills and other progestin-only options OR non-hormonal contraceptives. **Keeping a headache diary can help you understand what makes them better or worse and can help your clinician understand the possible causes of your headaches.**

May possibly continue using estrogen-containing pill as long but let your clinician know promptly

After a cycle or two have headaches clearly become worse (even if there are no neurovascular symptoms?)

YES

NO

Must **make change**
• to another method without estrogen
• to lower-estrogen pill **OR**
• stop pills completely
You need to be examined for other causes of headaches. Headaches can be treated. **Keeping a headache diary can help you understand what makes them better or worse and can help your clinician understand the possible causes of your headaches.**

May continue current combined pill or switch to lowest estrogen pill. You need to be examined for other causes of headaches. Headaches can be treated. **Keeping a headache diary can help you understand what makes them better or worse and can help your clinician understand the possible causes of your headaches.**

* If headaches are only in the pill-free (hormone-free) week, they may be due to estrogen withdrawal. Supplemental estrogen may help as may taking multiple cycles of pills with no break (see page 105) or use of a pill with a decreased hormone-free interval. The only pill with a decreased pill-free interval is Mircette.

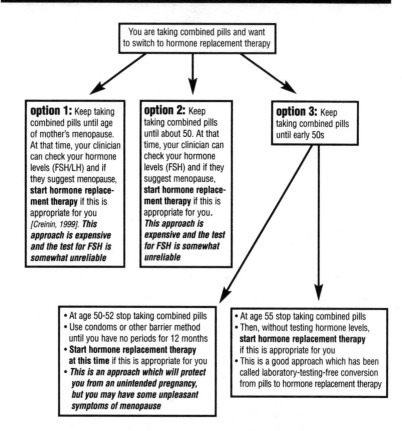

You are taking combined pills and want
to switch to hormone replacement therapy

option 1: Keep taking combined pills until age of mother's menopause. At that time, your clinician can check your hormone levels (FSH/LH) and if they suggest menopause, **start hormone replacement therapy** if this is appropriate for you *[Creinin, 1999].* ***This approach is expensive and the test for FSH is somewhat unreliable***

option 2: Keep taking combined pills until about 50. At that time, your clinician can check your hormone levels (FSH) and if they suggest menopause, **start hormone replacement therapy** if this is appropriate for you. ***This approach is expensive and the test for FSH is somewhat unreliable***

option 3: Keep taking combined pills until early 50s

- At age 50-52 stop taking combined pills
- Use condoms or other barrier method until you have no periods for 12 months
- **Start hormone replacement therapy at this time** if this is appropriate for you
- ***This is an approach which will protect you from an unintended pregnancy, but you may have some unpleasant symptoms of menopause***

- At age 55 stop taking combined pills
- Then, without testing hormone levels, **start hormone replacement therapy** if this is appropriate for you
- This is a good approach which has been called laboratory-testing-free conversion from pills to hormone replacement therapy

NOTE: *Not all women will want to or should go on hormone replacement therapy. This decision must be carefully reviewed by a woman and her clinician so that they can reach a decision together that is best for her.*

THE COLOR PAGES ARE ORGANIZED AS FOLLOWS:

PAGES 118-123: ....

There are many brands and types of oral contraceptive pills available. To help you become familiar with the different pills, we have included the following pages with color photos of pills. They are arranged in the following order:

• Progestin-only pills with no estrogen: Micronor, NOR-QD, and Ovrette

• Lowest estrogen pills with 20 micrograms (mcg) of estrogen (ethinyl estradiol): Alesse, Levlite, LoEstrin 1/20, and Mircette

• All of the 30- and 35-microgram pills

• All of the phasic pills (different levels of hormones in each pack)

• The highest estrogen pills, each of which has 50 micrograms of estrogen

There is an equal sign ($=$ or $||$) between pills which are chemically exactly the same.

The color and packaging of pills given out in clinics may differ from pills in pharmacies. The manufacturer of each pill is listed below each description.

PAGE 124: ....
Pills You Can Take as Emergency Contraception

PAGE 125: ....
Pill Warning Signals
The "ACHES" method tells you what to watch out for if you are taking pills and the problems that might be causing these symptoms.

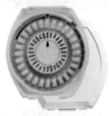 =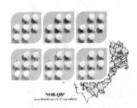

MICRONOR® TABLETS
28-DAY REGIMEN
(0.35 mg norethindrone)
Ortho-McNeil

NOR-QD® TABLETS
(0.35 mg norethindrone)
Watson

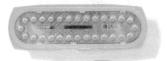

OVRETTE® TABLETS
(0.075 mg norgestrel)
Wyeth-Ayerst

COMBINED PILLS - 20 microgram PILLS

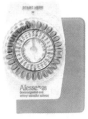 =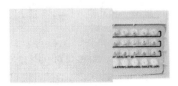

ALESSE - 28 TABLETS
(0.1 mg levonorgestrel/20 mcg ethinyl estradiol)
Wyeth-Ayerst

LEVLITE™ - 28 TABLETS
(0.1 mg levonorgestrel/20 mcg ethinyl estradiol)
Berlex

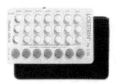

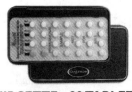

LOESTRIN® FE 1/20
(1 mg norethindrone acetate/20 mcg ethinyl
estradiol/75 mg ferrous fumarate [7d])
Parke-Davis

MIRCETTE - 28 TABLETS
(0.15 mg desogestrel/ 20 mcg ethinyl estradiol X 21 (white)/
placebo X 2 (green)/10 mcg ethinyl estradiol X 5 (yellow))
Organon

COMBINED PILLS - 30 microgram PILLS

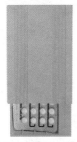

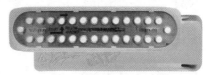

LO/OVRAL®-28 TABLETS
(0.3 mg norgestrel/30 mcg ethinyl estradiol)
Wyeth-Ayerst

=

LEVLEN® 28 TABLETS
(0.15 mg levonorgestrel/30 mcg ethinyl estradiol)
Berlex

||

||

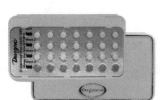

NORDETTE®-28 TABLETS
(0.15 mg levonorgestrel/30 mcg ethinyl estradiol)
Wyeth-Ayerst

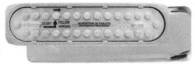

=

LEVORA TABLETS
(0.15 mg levonorgestrel/30 mcg ethinyl estradiol)
Watson

DESOGEN® 28 TABLETS
(0.15 mg desogestrel/30 mcg ethinyl estradiol)
Organon

=

**ORTHO-CEPT® TABLETS
28-DAY REGIMEN**
(0.15 mg desogestrel/30 mcg ethinyl estradiol)
Ortho-McNeil

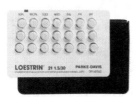

LOESTRIN® 21 1.5/30
(1.5 mg norethindrone acetate/ 30 mcg ethinyl estradiol)
Parke-Davis

119

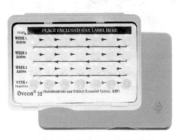

OVCON® 35 28-DAY
(0.4 mg norethindrone/35 mcg ethinyl estradiol)
Bristol-Myers

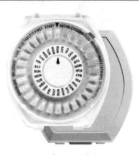

**ORTHO-CYCLEN®
28 TABLETS**
(0.25 mg norgestimate/35 mcg ethinyl estradiol)
Ortho-McNeil

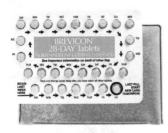

=

**BREVICON®
28-DAY TABLETS
Also available:
BREVICON® 21-DAY TABLETS**
(0.5 mg norethindrone/35 mcg ethinyl estradiol)
Watson

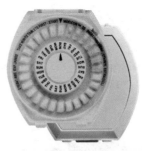

**MODICON® TABLETS
28-DAY REGIMEN**
(0.5 mg norethindrone/35 mcg ethinyl estradiol)
Ortho-McNeil

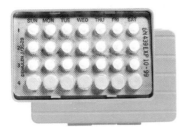

=

DEMULEN® 1/35-28
(1 mg ethynodiol diacetate/35 mcg ethinyl estradiol)
Searle

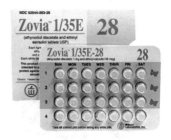

ZOVIA® 1/35E–28
(1 mg ethynodiol diacetate/35 mcg ethinyl estradiol)
Watson

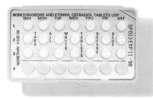

=

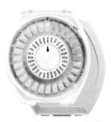

NORETHIN 1/35E–28
(1 mg norethindrone/35 mcg ethinyl estradiol)
Roberts

‖

ORTHO-NOVUM® 1/35
28 TABLETS
(1 mg norethindrone/35 mcg ethinyl estradiol)
Ortho-McNeil

‖

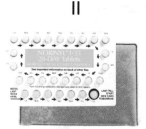

=

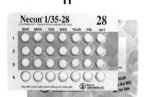

NORINYL® 1+35 28-DAY TABLETS
(1 mg norethindrone/35 mcg ethinyl estradiol)
Watson

NECON 1/35-28
(1 mg norethindrone/35 mcg ethinyl estradiol)
Watson

COMBINED PILLS - PHASIC PILLS

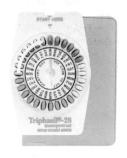

=

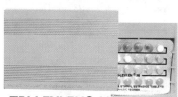

TRI-LEVLEN® 28 TABLETS
(levonorgestrel/ethinyl estradiol–triphasic regimen)
0.050 mg/30 mcg (6d), 0.075 mg/40 mcg (5d),
0.125 mg/30 mcg (10d)
Berlex

‖

TRIVORA®
(levonorgestrel/ethinyl estradiol–triphasic regimen)
0.050 mg/30 mcg (6d), 0.075 mg/40 mcg (5d),
0.125 mg/30 mcg (10d)
Watson

TRIPHASIL®-28 TABLETS
(levonorgestrel/ethinyl estradiol–triphasic regimen)
0.050 mg/30 mcg (6d), 0.075 mg/40 mcg (5d),
0.125 mg/30 mcg (10d)
Wyeth-Ayerst

=

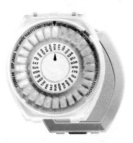

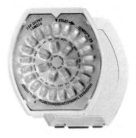

ORTHO-NOVUM® 10/11
28 TABLETS
(norethindrone/ethinyl estradiol)
0.5 mg/35 mcg (10d), 1 mg/35 mcg (11d)
Ortho-McNeil

JENEST 28 TABLETS
(norethindrone/ethinyl estradiol)
0.5 mg/35 mcg (7d), 1 mg/35 mcg (14d)
Organon

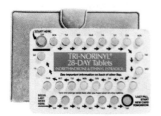

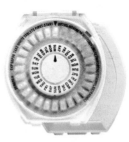

TRI-NORINYL®
28-DAY TABLETS
(norethindrone/ethinyl estradiol)
0.5 mg/35 mcg (7d), 1 mg/35 mcg (9d),
0.5 mg/35 mcg (5d)
Watson

ORTHO-NOVUM® 7/7/7
28 TABLETS
(norethindrone/ethinyl estradiol)
0.5 mg/35 mcg (7d), 0.75 mg/35 mcg (7d),
1 mg/35 mcg (7d)
Ortho-McNeil

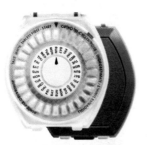

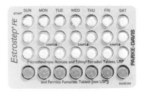

ORTHO TRI-CYCLEN®
28 TABLETS
(norgestimate/ethinyl estradiol)
0.18 mg/35 mcg (7d), 0.215 mg/35 mcg (7d),
0.25 mg/35 mcg (7d)
Ortho-McNeil

ESTROSTEP® FE
28 TABLETS
(norethindrone acetate/ethinyl estradiol)
1 mg/20 mcg (5d), 1 mg/30 mcg (7d),
1 mg/35 mcg (9d), 75 mg ferrous fumarate (7d)
Parke-Davis

122

COMBINED PILLS – 50 microgram PILLS

Pills with 50 micrograms of mestranol are not as strong as pills with 50 micrograms of ethinyl estradiol

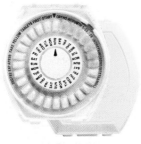

=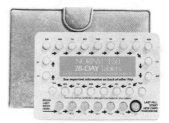

NORINYL® 1+50
28-DAY TABLETS
(1 mg norethindrone/50 mcg mestranol)
Watson

ORTHO-NOVUM® 1/50
28 TABLETS
(1 mg norethindrone/50 mcg mestranol)
Ortho-McNeil

‖

NECON 1/50
28-DAY TABLETS
(1 mg norethindrone/50 mcg mestranol)
Watson

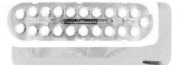

OVRAL - 21 TABLETS
(0.5 mg norgestrel/50 mcg ethinyl estradiol)
Wyeth-Ayerst

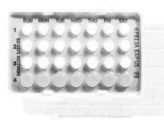

DEMULEN® 1/50-28
(1 mg ethynodiol diacetate/50 mcg ethinyl estradiol)
Watson

‖

ZOVIA® 1/50E–21 and 28
(1 mg ethynodiol diacetate/50 mcg ethinyl estradiol)
Watson

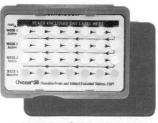

OVCON® 50 28-DAY
(1 mg norethindrone/50 mcg ethinyl estradiol)
Bristol-Myers

123

PILLS AS EMERGENCY CONTRACEPTIVES:
2 Different Approaches: Combined Pills OR Progestin-Only Pills

COMBINED ORAL CONTRACEPTIVES:

2 + 2 pills
12 hours apart

Preven *(blue pills)* **OR**
Ovral *(white pills)*
(Preven and Ovral are NOT carried
in all pharmacies. Check in advance.)

PREVEN
First pills marketed as
emergency contraceptives.
2 pills within 72 hours of unprotected sex;
2 pills 12 hours later
Call 1-888-PREVEN2

OR OVRAL

4 + 4 pills
12 hours apart

Lo-Ovral *(white pills)*,
Levora *(white pills)* **OR**
Levlen, OR
Nordette *(light orange pills)* **OR**
Triphasil *(yellow pills)*,
Trilevlen *(yellow pills)* **OR**
Trivora *(pink pills)*

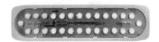

LO/OVRAL®-28 TABLETS
(0.3 mg norgestrel/30 mcg ethinyl estradiol)

OR ANY OF THE PILLS
LISTED TO THE LEFT

5 + 5 pills
12 hours apart

Alesse *(pink pills)* **OR**
Levlite *(pink pills)*

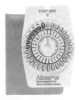

ALESSE -28 TABLETS
(0.1 mg levonorgestrel/20 mcg ethinyl estradiol)

OR LEVLITE

PROGESTIN-ONLY PILLS:

1 + 1 pill
12 hours apart

PLAN B

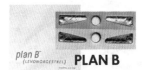

plan B™
(LEVONORGESTREL) **PLAN B**

20 + 20 pills
12 hours apart

Ovrette *(yellow pills)*

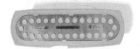

OR OVRETTE® TABLETS
(0.075 mg norgestrel)

124

PILL WARNING SIGNALS

Pills have been studied extensively and are very safe. However, very rarely pills lead to serious problems. Here are the warning signals to watch out for while using pills. These warning signals spell out the word **ACHES**. If you have one of these symptoms, it may or may not be related to pill use. You need to check with your clinician as soon as possible. The problems that could possibly be related to using pills are as follows:

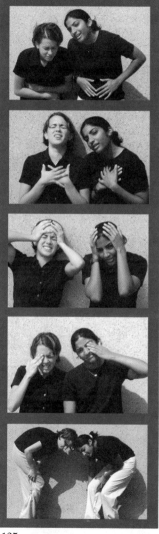

ABDOMINAL PAIN
• Blood clot in the pelvis or liver
• Liver tumor or gall bladder disease
• Pancreas inflammation

CHEST PAIN
• Blood clot in the lungs
• Heart attack
• Angina (heart pain)
• Breast lump

HEADACHES
• Stroke
• Migraine headache with neurological problems (blurred vision, spots, zigzag lines, weakness, difficulty speaking)
• Other headaches caused by pills
• High blood pressure

EYE PROBLEMS
• Stroke
• Blurred vision, double vision, or loss of vision
• Migraine headache with neurological problems (blurred vision, spots, zigzag lines)
• Blood clots in the eyes
• Change in shape of cornea (contacts don't fit)

SEVERE LEG PAIN
• Inflammation and blood clots of a vein in the leg
• Severe blood clots in the leg

You should also return to the clinic if you develop severe mood swings or depression, become jaundiced (yellow-colored skin), miss 2 periods or have signs of pregnancy.

WHAT IS DEPO-PROVERA?

A progestin-only injection which a woman gets from her clinician on schedule once every 3 months. It is often effective for more than 13 weeks. A woman usually gets the injection in the upper arm or buttock.

HOW EFFECTIVE IS DEPO-PROVERA?

Perfect-use failure rate in first year: Less than 0.3%
Typical-use failure rate in first year: 0.3% (Of every 1,000 women who use this method, 3 will become pregnant in first year)

[Trussell J, Contraceptive Technology, 1998]

HOW MUCH DOES DEPO-PROVERA COST?

	Managed care setting	*Public provider setting*
Drug	$30/injection	$30/injection
Office visit	$ 38/visit	$16.56/visit

[Trussell, 1995; Smith, 1993]

HOW DOES DEPO-PROVERA WORK?

The progestin stops ovulation so that an egg is not released; makes cervical mucus thicker so that sperm cannot get through; and changes the lining of the uterus so that implantation of the fertilized egg in the uterine wall does not occur.

WHAT ARE THE ADVANTAGES OF DEPO-PROVERA?

Menstrual:
- Possible improvement in endometriosis
- Decreased cramps and pain during periods and during ovulation
- Decreased blood loss during periods; it is normal for some women to gradually stop having periods altogether
- Less anemia (low blood count often caused by a low iron level)

Sexual/psychological:
- Sex may be enjoyed more because less fear of pregnancy

Cancers, tumors, and masses:
- Possible reduced risk for ovarian and endometrial uterine cancer

Other:
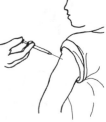
- Can prevent ectopic pregnancies
- Nothing to take each day or use at the time of sex
- Only needs to be remembered 4 times a year
- Privacy. No one has to know a woman is using this method
- Extremely effective. Single decision leads to 3 months of contraception
- Remains effective if woman returns a week or two late for shot
- May be "forgiving" even if woman is much *more* than 2 weeks late. The average first ovulation is about 10 months after a woman's last shot. The problem is that a woman cannot count on this delay in ovulation. In some women ovulation returns quickly, so it is important to go back **ON TIME** for your shots
- Unlike combined pills, Depo-Provera is not less effective if you take medicines that affect the liver
- Even safer than combined pills (no blood clotting problems)

- May be used by some women who cannot take estrogen, such as women who have had severe blood clots (NOTE: Package insert says differently)
- Can be used throughout the reproductive years. No rest periods needed
- Reversible, but return of fertility tends to take longer than other hormonal methods (see page 131)
- Possible decreased risk of symptomatic pelvic inflammatory disease (PID)
- Possible decreased risk of sickle cell crises from sickle cell anemia and grand mal seizures from epilepsy
- May be used by nursing mothers. Progestin-only contraception does not decrease and may even increase the amount of mother's milk. Babies whose mothers use Depo-Provera while breastfeeding develop normally both physically and mentally in the first year of life

WHAT ARE THE DISADVANTAGES OF DEPO-PROVERA?

Menstrual:
- May lead to unwanted changes in menstrual cycle: irregular bleeding, missed periods or no periods (common); heavy bleeding (rare). It is a good idea to be examined by a clinician if you are concerned (go to **www.managingcontraception.com** for more information)
- Irregular bleeding from another cause may be incorrectly linked to Depo-Provera
- Less than 1/3 of women report normal periods during first year of use
- Takes many months for some women to stop having periods altogether
- PMS symptoms may worsen (but are more likely to improve)

Sexual/psychological:
- Sex may be enjoyed less because some women have decreased sex drive, vaginal lubrication, or orgasms
- Increased days of spotting may interfere with sex for some women
- Depression may get worse (but more likely to get better); anxiety, mood changes, or fatigue may occur

Cancers, tumors, and masses: None
Other:
- Must use condoms if at risk for sexually transmitted infections, including HIV/AIDS
- Must return every 3 months for injection (can be hard for some women to remember)
- Expensive in some health-care settings
- May have a negative effect on bone growth in teens; may increase risk of osteoporosis (brittle bones)
- Increased appetite and/or weight gain; women gain several pounds per year on average (go to **www.managingcontraception.com** for details on weight gain and specific ways of avoiding this problem)
- It takes an average of 10 months for fertility to return after the last shot, making it hard to plan pregnancy exactly
- Estrogen is suppressed in some women
- Severe headaches may occur
- Increase in LDL (bad cholesterol) and decrease in HDL (good cholesterol) in some studies
- Higher dose of progestin than combined pills, minipills or Norplant
- Rarely a woman is allergic to Depo-Provera, but if she is the effects of the shot cannot be stopped once it is given. Such a woman may need anti-allergy medicine for several days to months
- *Rare:* excessive weight gain, severe depression, severe allergic reaction

WHAT ARE THE RISKS OF DEPO-PROVERA?
- Rare: excessive weight gain
- Rare: severe depression (on average there is no change in women using Depo-Provera)
- Rare: severe allergic reactions. It may be a good idea to wait in or near the clinic for 20 minutes after your first injection

IS DEPO-PROVERA THE RIGHT METHOD FOR ME?

Ask yourself the questions below. If you answer NO to ALL of the questions, then you CAN probably use Depo-Provera. If you answer YES to a question below, follow the instructions.

1. Do you think you might be pregnant?

☐ No   ☐ Yes   If yes, you need to find out if you are pregnant. Use condoms or spermicide until you and your clinician are reasonably sure that you are not pregnant. Then you may start Depo-Provera.

2. Do you plan to become pregnant in the next year?

☐ No   ☐ Yes   If yes, use another method that may cause less delay in return of fertility after discontinuing that method.

3. Are you breastfeeding a baby less than 6 weeks old? (p. 129)

☐ No   ☐ Yes   If yes, you can get your first shot before you leave the hospital, if your milk flow has been established. There is no evidence that Depo-Provera has a negative effect on a nursing newborn baby or on the quality or amount of breast milk that is produced. There is some controversy about providing Depo-Provera prior to 6 weeks after birth.

4. Do you have or have you had problems with your heart or blood vessels? If so, what problems?

☐ No   ☐ Yes   If yes, you cannot use Depo-Provera if you have had a heart attack, stroke, heart disease from blocked arteries, severe high blood pressure, diabetes for more than 20 years, damage to your vision, kidneys, or nervous system caused by diabetes. Your provider can help you choose another effective method.

5. Do you have or have you ever had breast cancer?

☐ No   ☐ Yes   If yes, you cannot use Depo-Provera. Your clinician can help you choose another method without hormones.

6. Do you have jaundice, severe cirrhosis of the liver or a liver infection or tumor? (Are your eyes or skin unusually yellow?)

☐ No   ☐ Yes   If yes, get a physical exam. If you have a serious liver disease (jaundice, painful or enlarged liver, hepatitis, liver tumor), you cannot use Depo-Provera and need to be treated for the liver problem. Your clinician can help you choose another method without hormones.

7. Do you have vaginal bleeding that is unusual for you?

☐ No   ☐ Yes   If yes, and if you have vaginal bleeding that may be from another already-diagnosed medical problem, you may be able to use Depo-Provera. Any problem should be assessed by your clinician and a decision made about its treatment.

8. Are you 30-35 or older AND do you definitely want a pregnancy in the future?

☐ No   ☐ Yes   If yes, strongly consider a different contraceptive because you may not get your period for a long time (10 months on average or larger) after you stop using Depo-Provera.

WHO CAN USE DEPO-PROVERA INJECTIONS?
Women who:
- Want privacy, high level of effectiveness, convenience
- Have a reason not to use estrogen
- Can return every 3 months
- Will use condoms if at risk of infection
- Have just given birth (regardless of breastfeeding) or have just had an abortion
- Prefer to take medicine as a shot
- Are using a medicine that affects the liver (which makes other hormonal contraceptives less effective)
- Have sickle cell disease, seizures, endometriosis, PMS symptoms, or fibroids
- Have difficulty using other methods that require remembering to do something every day such as taking a pill

What About Adolescents?
- Extremely effective. Increased use of Depo-Provera by teens is credited with much of the recent drop in teenage pregnancies in the United States
- Confidential (see page 18 for information on laws in your state)
- Decreased pain during periods, PMS, endometriosis and pelvic inflammatory disease (PID)
- May cause weight gain; causes irregular periods, both of which may be unacceptable to teens
- Many teens stop using it because they have to come back to the clinic 4 times a year
- Long-term effect on bones not fully understood (may, temporarily, decrease bone growth in adolescents) *[Cromer, 1996]*

HOW DO I START THE METHOD?
- Women having periods may start Depo-Provera shots on the first day of bleeding (best approach), **OR** any of the first 5 days after bleeding starts **OR** any time they are not pregnant
- Use a backup method for 7 days after your first shot if it is not given during the first 5 days of bleeding. Some clinics recommend using a backup contraceptive the first 7 days after the first shot no matter when it is started
- *If you have just given birth and are breastfeeding, it is best to start Depo-Provera after your breast milk supply has been established. There is a debate among experts about whether it is OK to start Depo-Provera right after a woman has given birth. Bleeding after giving birth is a problem for some women and rarely Depo-Provera might increase bleeding*
- If you are not breastfeeding, it is OK to start Depo-Provera any time after giving birth, as soon as you want it. There is no need to wait until your periods start again. If it has been 6 weeks or more since you have given birth, you must be reasonably sure you are not pregnant when starting Depo-Provera
- If you have had a miscarriage or an abortion, it is OK to start Depo-Provera in the first 5 days after the miscarriage or abortion. After 5 days, it is OK to start as long as you are reasonably sure you are not pregnant
- If you are stopping another method, you can start Depo-Provera right away. For example, there is no need to wait for your period after using pills, Norplant, or an IUD. It is a good idea to use a backup method for 7 days after your first shot, though, if it was not given within the first 5 days of your period

WHAT GUIDELINES DO I NEED TO FOLLOW?
- Do not rub the area where shot is given for first few hours
- Expect irregular bleeding. This usually decreases over time.
  After 6-12 months there will probably be very little or no vaginal bleeding (i.e., no periods)
- You may also have very light bleeding or no bleeding at all. This is normal and not harmful
- Return at any time if the bleeding pattern is bothersome. Medicines are available that may make the bleeding pattern more acceptable to you   129

- Weight gain is common. The average weight gain is 3 to 4.5 pounds in the first year. Eating less and exercising more are the best two ways to solve this problem (see **www.managingcontraception.com**)
- Return in 11 or 12 weeks for next injection
- If it has been more than 13 weeks since your last shot, avoid intercourse or use condoms until your next shot
- Return just as soon as you realize you are late for your shot; you may still be able to get an injection of Depo-Provera right away
- Serious problems from Depo-Provera are rare. Return to your clinic if you have: pus, prolonged pain, or bleeding from the injection site, repeated, very painful headaches; heavy bleeding; depression; severe lower abdominal pain (may be a sign of pregnancy)
- The effects of Depo-Provera on your bones are not fully understood; calcium, exercise and not smoking are good for your bones whether or not you are on Depo-Provera (see **www.managingcontraception.com**)
- Drug or alcohol use may reduce the effectiveness of Depo-Provera. For example, being drunk or high may increase the risk of returning late for an injection or missing an injection completely, and is associated with failure to use condoms during intercourse when there is a risk for infections

DO I NEED TO CONSULT MY CLINICIAN? ASK YOURSELF:

Following are important questions to help you evaluate your use of Depo-Provera. If you answer "yes" to any question, talk to your clinician to figure out the best solution for you.

☐ Am I having spotting, irregular bleeding, or heavy bleeding that is concerning me?
☐ Have I had significant pain, bleeding or pus at the injection site?
☐ Do I have breast tenderness or have I felt a breast lump?
☐ Have I felt depressed or had major mood changes?
☐ Have I been less interested in sex or do I enjoy sex less?
☐ Have I gained 5 pounds or more?
☐ Do I have repeated or very severe headaches?
☐ Have I had severe lower abdominal pain, nausea or vomiting?
☐ Do I think I may be pregnant?
☐ Do I have any questions I would like to ask my clinician?

WHAT HAPPENS IF:

I gain weight? Carefully watch calories, exercise more and eat less if you start to gain weight. **Stop using Depo-Provera if the weight gain is unacceptable to you. Talk to your clinician about trying another method.**

I have irregular bleeding? Irregular bleeding is normal and is usually not harmful. If you have no reason to avoid estrogen, combined pills may help make bleeding more regular. Any of the low-dose pills (20 microgram pills: Alesse, LoEstrin 1/20, or Mircette), oral estrogen, or a medicine like ibuprofen may help. Usually combined pills are given for one cycle or less. If 1 week to 1 month of pills does not improve or solve the problem, more than one cycle of pills may be given.

I have heavy bleeding? If you are worried, go to your clinician to have the bleeding checked. You may need to have blood tests done. If you are anemic (low blood count), you may need to eat foods that have iron in them or take iron pills. It may also help to take a low-dose combined pill, estrogen supplements, or a medicine like ibuprofen to help control the bleeding. You and your clinician can decide on the best approach for you.

I don't get periods? Not getting your period is a normal effect of Depo-Provera and is not harmful. Periods usually become light and you are likely to have no periods at the longer you continue to use Depo-Provera.

I get depressed? It is important to go to your clinician to have the depression evaluated. The depression may not be caused by the Depo-Provera. If you are extremely depressed or suicidal, you need to seek help immediately. Your clinician can respond appropriately to your depression or direct you to help right away. Stop Depo-Provera if it looks like the depression is related to it (the depression should get better as time goes on, but may last 3 or more months after your last shot). If you stop Depo-Provera, be sure to use another method if you want to avoid pregnancy.

I have an allergic reaction? If it is a mild reaction, your clinician needs to stop giving you injections and you may take a medicine like Benedryl to stop the reaction. Even though Depo-Provera stays in your body for an average of 10 months, the allergic reaction should get better in a week after your shot. Although severe allergic reactions are rare, it may be a good idea for you to wait in the clinic for 20 minutes after your shot to make sure you do not have a reaction. If it is severe, it needs immediate treatment.

I have vaginal dryness? Depo-Provera causes your cervical mucus to get thick and decreases the amount of estrogen in you body. Both of these can make your vagina feel dry. Usually it helps to use a water-based lubricant like K-Y Jelly or Wet when you have sex (see page 49 for suggestions).

I have pain where I got the injection? Some discomfort at injection site is normal. Do not rub the area where you got the shot. This can make the pain worse and may make Depo-Provera less effective in the third month of the shot. You can take a medicine like ibuprofen to help pain and swelling. Go back to your clinician if the area gets infected (this is rare).

I come back more than 13 weeks after my last injection? (see page 132)

I want to switch from Depo-Provera to combined pills? (see page 133)

I want to stop Depo-Provera because I am approaching menopause? If and when ovulation starts varies from woman to woman. You might take a low-dose combined pill estrogen supplement for 2-3 years before anticipated age of menopause if you have no reason to avoid estrogen (see page 134).

FERTILITY AFTER USE
• Eventual return of fertility is excellent after using Depo-Provera
• Average of 10 months delay in return of ovulation. More than 90% of women become pregnant within 2 years of stopping Depo-Provera. Because it may take more than 1 year for fertility to return, women over 30-35 years old who know they will want to get pregnant after stopping contraception, especially if over 35 years old, would be wise to consider a different method of birth control

You are late for your next Depo-Provera shot

This can be a difficult issue for clinicians and women on Depo-Provera

/ You are late (more than 13 weeks) & want your next Depo-Provera shot

Note: If you are having a definite period, you can get a Depo-Provera shot at this time

I have not had sexual intercourse since 13 weeks after my last shot

- You can get your next shot immediately. Use backup method for 7 days
- Pregnancy test optional
- Your clinician will need to document your sexual history carefully on your chart

I HAVE HAD SEXUAL INTERCOURSE since 13 weeks after last shot

Was all sexual intercourse PROTECTED since 13 weeks after last shot?

YES: You can get your next shot immediately if pregnancy test is negative. Your clinician will need to document your sexual history carefully on your chart

Did you have UNPROTECTED sexual intercourse since 13 weeks after last shot?

YES and all unprotected intercourse was within past 72 hours

Take emergency contraceptive pills; know that they are not 100% effective, AND

- Take Depo-Provera shot immediately
- Use backup contraception for 7 days
- Your clinician will need to document your sexual history carefully on your chart and have you initial it

YES and unprotected intercourse was BOTH within past 72 hours AND more than 72 hours ago

If negative pregnancy test:
- Take emergency contraceptive pills and know that they are not 100% effective before or after 72 hours and will not have an effect on an established pregnancy
- Use backup contraception for 2 weeks, then return to clinic

YES: and all unprotected intercourse was MORE than 72 hours ago

If pregnancy test is negative: avoid intercourse or use backup contraceptive for 2 weeks then return to clinic

- 2 weeks later repeat pregnancy test
- If negative you can get your Depo-Provera shot
- Use backup contraception for 7 days
- Your clinician will need to document your sexual history carefully on your chart and have you initial it

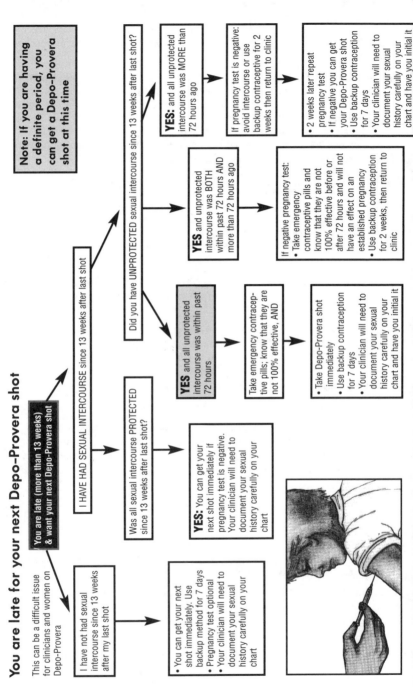

You want to switch from Depo-Provera to Combined Pills

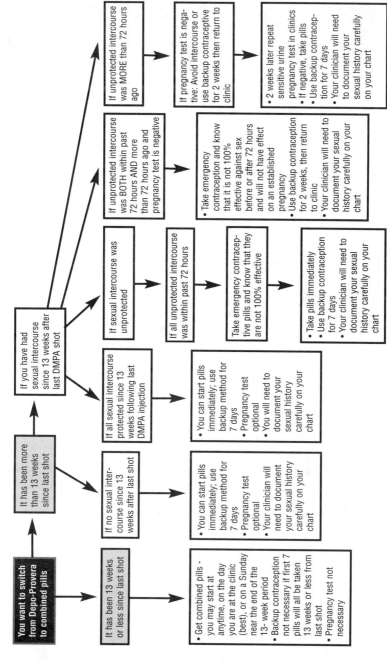

You want to switch from Depo-Provera to combined pills

It has been 13 weeks or less since last shot

- Get combined pills - you may start at anytime, on the day you are at the clinic (best), or on a Sunday near the end of the 13-week period
- Backup contraception not necessary if first 7 pills will all be taken 13 weeks or less from last shot
- Pregnancy test not necessary

It has been more than 13 weeks since last shot

If no sexual intercourse since 13 weeks after last shot

- You can start pills immediately; use backup method for 7 days
- Pregnancy test optional
- Your clinician will need to document your sexual history carefully on your chart

If you have had sexual intercourse since 13 weeks after last DMPA shot

If all sexual intercourse protected since 13 weeks following last DMPA injection

- You can start pills immediately; use backup method for 7 days
- Pregnancy test optional
- You will need to document your sexual history carefully on your chart

If sexual intercourse was unprotected

If all unprotected intercourse was within past 72 hours

Take emergency contraceptive pills and know that they are not 100% effective

- Take pills immediately
- Use backup contraception for 7 days
- Your clinician will need to document your sexual history carefully on your chart

If unprotected intercourse was BOTH within past 72 hours AND more than 72 hours ago and pregnancy test is negative

- Take emergency contraception and know that it is not 100% effective against sex before or after 72 hours and will not have effect on an established pregnancy
- Use backup contraception for 2 weeks, then return to clinic
- Your clinician will need to document your sexual history carefully on your chart

If unprotected intercourse was MORE than 72 hours ago

If pregnancy test is negative: Avoid intercourse or use backup contraceptive for 2 weeks then return to clinic

- 2 weeks later repeat sensitive urine pregnancy test in clinics
- If negative, take pills
- Use backup contraception for 7 days
- Your clinician will need to document your sexual history carefully on your chart

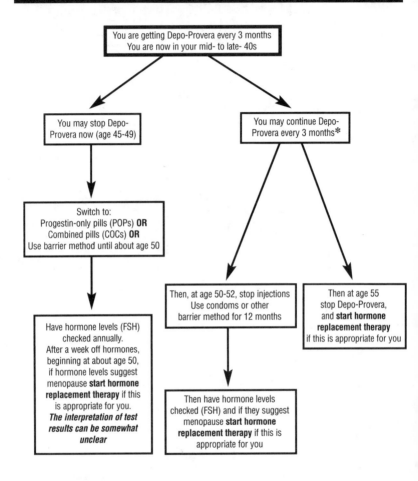

You are getting Depo-Provera every 3 months
You are now in your mid- to late- 40s

You may stop Depo-Provera now (age 45-49)

You may continue Depo-Provera every 3 months*

Switch to:
Progestin-only pills (POPs) **OR**
Combined pills (COCs) **OR**
Use barrier method until about age 50

Then, at age 50-52, stop injections
Use condoms or other barrier method for 12 months

Then at age 55 stop Depo-Provera, and **start hormone replacement therapy** if this is appropriate for you

Have hormone levels (FSH) checked annually.
After a week off hormones, beginning at about age 50, if hormone levels suggest menopause **start hormone replacement therapy** if this is appropriate for you.
The interpretation of test results can be somewhat unclear

Then have hormone levels checked (FSH) and if they suggest menopause **start hormone replacement therapy** if this is appropriate for you

* Depo-Provera causes natural estrogen levels in your body to go down. For this reason, some experts say it is a good idea for women in their 40s who have been using Depo-Provera for a long time to take estrogen supplements. Then, when they are 55 years old, they can switch to hormone replacement therapy. This approach is simple and expensive tests are not needed. *[Kaunitz, 1998]*

CHAPTER 29

Combined Injections
www.conrad.org

WHAT ARE COMBINED INJECTIONS?
An injection of estrogen and progestin that you get once a month. Available starting June 2000 in the USA under the name of Lunelle. Do not confuse this with the every-three-month injections of Depo-Provera.

HOW EFFECTIVE ARE COMBINED INJECTIONS?
Perfect-use failure rate in first year: 0.2 - 0.4% (2-4 women per 1000 using it for one year would get pregnant)
Typical-use failure rate in first year: Same

HOW DO COMBINED INJECTIONS WORK?
Stops ovulation and estrogen keeps the lining of the uterus stable.

COST: Unknown; not available in the U.S.A.

WHAT ARE THE ADVANTAGES OF COMBINED INJECTIONS?
Menstrual: Compared to Depo-Provera, more regular bleeding pattern and women keep
    normal estrogen levels
Sexual/ psychological:
- Single shot gives 1 month of contraception; nothing to do at time of intercourse
- Private and confidential
- Fertility comes back quickly (average of 3 months)
Cancers, tumors, and masses:
- Not enough long-term research to know for sure
- No known increased risk of breast cancer
Other:
- Very effective

WHAT ARE THE DISADVANTAGES OF COMBINED INJECTIONS?
Menstrual: Irregular periods (less of a problem than with Depo-Provera)
Sexual/psychological:
- Must return to clinic every 30 days, unless you learn how to inject yourself and your clinician is willing to provide you with 6-12 injections
- You may not like repeated injections
- Medicine cannot be reverted once shot is given
Cancers, tumors, and masses: Not enough long-term research to know for sure
Other:
- Expensive in some clinics
- Not ideal for breastfeeding women
- Breast tenderness

WHO CAN USE COMBINED INJECTIONS?
Women who:
- Can use combined pills
- Want highly effective reversible method
- Want to have a child within 1-2 years
- Do not want to take pills every day

What About Adolescents? Requires visits every month, which may be difficult for teens.   135

CHAPTER 30

Contraceptive Implants: Norplant
www.managingcontraception.com or 1-800-760-9030

WHAT IS NORPLANT?

6 soft flexible plastic rods (34 millimeters long x 2.4 millimeters wide) that contain the hormone **levonorgestrel** (which is previously discussed as a part of birth control pills and one of the IUDs). A clinician inserts the rods in a woman's upper arm through minor surgery. This safe, effective contraceptive has never realized its potential for a number of complicated reasons.

HOW EFFECTIVE IS NORPLANT?

Perfect-use failure rate in first year: 0.05% (1 out of every 2000 women using Norplant will get pregnant in the first year of use)

Typical-user failure rate in first year: 0.05%

Total failure rate after 5 years: 1.5% (women who weigh 131 to 153 pounds)
2.4% (women who weigh more than 154 pounds)
[Trussell J, Contraceptive Technology, 1998]

Evidence is increasing that Norplant implants remain effective for more than 5 years. Ask your clinician.

HOW DOES NORPLANT WORK?

Norplant starts working within 72 hours of insertion. It makes cervical mucus thicker, which stops sperm from going into the uterus. It also reduces or stops ovulation. Women who use Norplant do not ovulate very often, especially in the first 2 years of using Norplant. Norplant also keeps the lining of the uterus thin, so that implantation of the fertilized egg does not occur.

WILL NORPLANT DECREASE THE AMOUNT OF ESTROGEN IN MY BODY?

Norplant does not cause estrogen levels in a woman's body to decrease the way Depo-Provera sometimes does. In studies, the levels of estrogen in women using Norplant was similar to the levels of estrogen in women not using contraception.

HOW MUCH DOES NORPLANT COST?

	Managed care setting:	*Public provider setting:*
Implants	$365	$365.00*
Insertion	333	47.96
Removal	100	79.64

[Trussell, 1995; Smith, 1993]

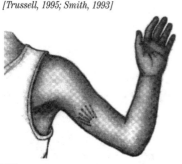

* The Norplant Foundation provides free Norplant insertion and help with Norplant removal for women who qualify:
1-800-760-9030

WHAT ARE THE ADVANTAGES OF NORPLANT?

Menstrual:
- Less blood loss during periods
- Less cramping or pain during periods; less pain from ovulation

Sexual/psychological:
- Reduced fear of pregnancy may increase enjoyment of sex
- Depression and PMS may get better

Cancers, tumors, and masses:
- Risk of endometrial cancer and/or ovarian cancer may be decreased

Other:
- Highly effective. Single decision and a 10 to 15 minute procedure may lead to long-term contraception
- Many women (88%) keep using Norplant after the first year
- Reduced risk of ectopic pregnancy*
- Decrease in blood loss leading to anemia (even in most women who have it taken out because of bleeding)
- Reccuring headaches, occasional headaches and migraines may get better
- Very low dose of progestin and no estrogen
- May be used by some women who cannot take estrogen

*NOTE: Ectopic pregnancies in women who use Norplant are rare. Norplant offers significant protection against pregnancy outside the uterus (ectopic pregnancy), but it could still occur. When pregnancy does occur in a woman using Norplant, 1 pregnancy in every 6 is ectopic.

WHAT ARE THE DISADVANTAGES OF NORPLANT? (also see page 138)

Menstrual:
- No periods, irregular bleeding, spotting, very light periods
- Because of hormone changes, the ovaries may get enlarged because eggs are not being released (happens in 20% of Norplant users). Most of the time, this goes away on its own in 1-3 months and is not a problem. See your clinician if you have any pain or swelling in the lower abdomen

Sexual/psychological: Possible mood changes; worsening depression, anxiety, or irritability
Cancers, tumors, and masses: None
Other:
- Does not protect against HIV or STIs
- You have to go to a clinic to get Norplant out and taking it out might be difficult (if it was poorly inserted or if the person taking the implants out is inexperienced)
- May have a problem finding someone trained and willing to remove implants
- Irregular bleeding with more days of bleeding (but less blood loss); by the 5th year two thirds of women have regular cycles
- Headaches may become worse (second most common reason for removal)
- Breast tenderness
- Weight gain or loss (average gain 5 pounds over 5 years, which is close to the average among women in their early to mid-reproductive years)
- You might be able to see the Norplant implants under the skin or the skin over it may get darker
- Hair growth or loss
- Pain during or few days after insertion or removal
- Itching at insertion site
- Norplant is less effective if you take drugs that affect the liver (e.g., rifampicin, griseofulvin and most antiseizure medicines)
- Initial cost high

WHAT ARE THE RISKS OF NORPLANT?

- Difficult removal or damage to nerve in arm during removal of implants that are very deep
- Severe headaches with blurred vision (it has not been proven that these headaches are caused by Norplant, but an association has been reported)
- Rare, abnormal weight gain
- Large painful ovarian cysts. They usually go away without treatment in 1 to 2 months *[Fraser, 1997]*
- Allergy to the hormone levonorgestrel (rare)
- Irritation or infection at the place where Norplant implants are inserted or removed.
- Rarely, an implant may come out on its own

Top twenty medical complaints from Norplant users* (Note: These are complaints. It does not necessarily mean that these problems were caused by a woman's Norplant implants)

Problem/Complaint	Average number of times women had this problem per year
Headache	12.8
Whitish vaginal discharge	12.6
Pelvic pain	7.3
Weight gain	5.4
General itching	5.1
Nervousness	4.3
Dizziness	4.1
Infection of the cervix	4.0
Breast pain	3.9
Yeast infection	3.3
Benign breast lump	2.8
Cervical lesion	2.7
Acne	2.7
Nausea	2.6
Weakness	2.4
Pain at implant site	2.2
Irritation at implant site	2.1
Hair Loss	1.9
Tiredness	1.8
Painful or difficult urination	1.7

*Sivin I, Viegas OAC, et al. Clinical performance of a new two-rod levonorgestrel contraceptive implant: a three-year randomized study with Norplant implants as controls. Contraception 1997;55:80.

WHO CAN USE NORPLANT?

Women who:

- Want an effective, long-term contraceptive
- Are young, do not have children; are at any age of the reproductive years
- Will use condoms if at risk of infection
- Have just given birth (breastfeeding or not breastfeeding)
- Are breastfeeding and are just leaving the hospital after birth or are returning for their first clinic visit after giving birth
- Have just had an abortion
- Are at any point in their cycle if it is certain that they are not pregnant

What About Adolescents? Norplant is a good option for adolescents. The continuation rate in teens using Norplant is higher than the continuation rate among teens using pills or Depo-Provera.

IS NORPLANT THE RIGHT METHOD FOR ME?

IMPORTANT: Norplant implants do not have estrogen. Many of the reasons a woman might not be able to take combined pills, which contain estrogen, do not apply to Norplant implants.

Ask yourself the questions below. If you answer NO to ALL of the questions, then you CAN probably use Norplant implants if you want. If you answer YES to a question below, follow the instructions. In some cases, you can still use Norplant implants.

1. Do you think you are pregnant?

☐ No   ☐ Yes If yes, you need to find out if you are pregnant. If you might be pregnant, check a pregnancy test or use condoms or spermicide until reasonably sure that you are not pregnant. Then you can start Norplant implants.

2. Do you have jaundice, cirrhosis of the liver, or a liver infection or tumor? (Are your eyes or skin unusually yellow?)

☐ No   ☐ Yes If yes, you need to have a physical exam. If you have a serious liver disease (jaundice, painful or enlarged liver, hepatitis, liver tumor), you cannot use Norplant implants and need to be treated for the liver problem. Your clinician can help you choose another method without hormones.

3. Do you have or have you ever had breast cancer?

☐ No   ☐ Yes If yes, you probably cannot use Norplant implants. Your clinician can help you choose a method without hormones.

4. Do you have vaginal bleeding that is unusual for you?

☐ No   ☐ Yes If yes, and you have unexplained vaginal bleeding that might be from pregnancy or another medical problem, you cannot use Norplant implants. You need to be diagnosed and treated for the medical problem. Your clinician can help you choose a method without hormones to use until the problem is diagnosed and treated. Then you can start using Norplant implants.

5. Are you taking medicine for seizures? Are you taking the antibiotics rifampin or griseofulvin?

☐ No   ☐ Yes If yes, and you are taking medicines for seizures or the antibiotics rifampin or griseofulvin, consistently use condoms or spermicide along with Norplant implants. If you prefer, or if you are on long-term treatment, your clinician can help you choose another effective method of contraception.

6. Have you just given birth and are breastfeeding, and do you want to have Norplant implants inserted before you leave the hospital?

☐ No   ☐ Yes If yes, you may be able to obtain the Norplant right away. Many experts disagree as to whether breastfeeding may be interfered with by immediate Norplant insertion. Many clinicians and hospitals, however, are willing to provide this service [IPPF, 1997; Anderson, 1997].

HOW DO I START THE METHOD?

- Norplant implants are put in under the skin of the upper arm during a minor surgical procedure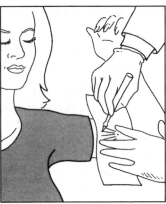
- In many cases, you may have Norplant put in on the same day in the clinic that you decide you want it. In other cases, you may have to make another appointment and come back to have Norplant put in
- First, your clinician will use a marker to trace a pattern on your arm where the implants will go (see picture to the right)
- Next she or he will numb the area using a local anesthetic that is injected with a needle under the skin where each of the implants will go
- Then, your clinician will make a small cut (1/4 inch) with a scalpel and will insert each of the implants with a special tool (see picture below)
- **You should not be able to feel anything except for slight pulling or tugging. Tell your clinician if you feel any pain or discomfort during the procedure and he or she will make the area more numb**
- After the implants are in, your clinician will cover the area with bandages. One bandage will be sticky and will hold the small cut together so it can heal. The other bandage will be a wrap that will put pressure on the area to make sure it does not bleed
- A medicine such as ibuprofen can help relieve pain you may have and hour or so after insertion

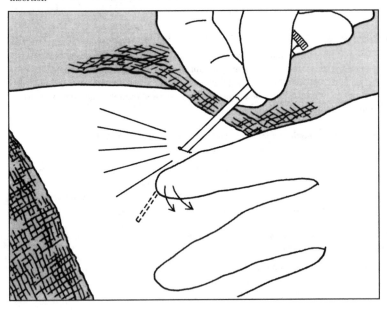

WHAT GUIDELINES DO I NEED TO FOLLOW?

- Keep the insertion area dry for 4 days
- See page 144 to see if and how long you need to use a backup contraceptive method
- Bandage wrap may be taken off in 1-2 days, but let the small adhesive bandage fall off by itself
- Expect irregular bleeding when using Norplant. If the bleeding is unacceptable, go back to the clinic because there are some things that may be done to improve it
- When implants are inserted, you should know where to go to have them taken out by a trained clinician AND you need to know that implants may be taken out for any reason. It is your decision
- Return to your clinician if you have any of these danger or warning signs:
  - Severe lower abdominal pain (ectopic pregnancy is rare but can occur and large ovarian cysts may need to be evaluated)
  - Very heavy bleeding during your period
  - Severe arm pain (soreness after the numbing wears off is normal)
  - Pus, redness, heat or bleeding where the implants were inserted (this might mean infection)
  - Part or all of an implant is pushed out
  - Severe headaches or blurred vision that get worse after Norplant insertion
  - Possible pregnancy (missed period after some regular cycles or nausea)
- Norplant slowly gets less effective after 5 years. If contraception is NOT needed, Norplant may be left in place. They are not dangerous to you if they stay in your arm. In some places Norplant implants are being left in place for more that 5 years. Low pregnancy rates have been found up to 7 years after insertion (research has not yet been published)
- If you want another set of implants, you can have the first set removed at the five-year point and the second set inserted at the same time, through the same incision

- **IMPORTANT:** If you choose Norplant, you must be able to get it taken out when you want it out. All clinicians that offer Norplant must have qualified staff that can put it in or take it out, or a referral system for taking it out. You may call the Norplant Foundation for names of clinicians who will take out implants and to get help with money for the procedure. **The number to call is: 1-800-760-9030.**

DO I NEED TO CONSULT MY CLINICIAN? ASK YOURSELF:

Following are important questions to help you evaluate your use of Norplant. If you answer "yes" to any question, talk to your clinician to figure out the best solution for you

- ☐ Have I had any changes in my menstrual cycle?
- ☐ Have I had a delayed menstrual period after a long interval of regular periods?
- ☐ Is the bleeding bothersome to me?
- ☐ Have I noticed any changes in color or pain level at the place Norplant was put in?
- ☐ Have I noticed breast tenderness or pain?
- ☐ Do I have severe headaches?
- ☐ Have I had any allergic reaction or irritation?
- ☐ Have I had persistent arm pain, pus, bleeding or partial expulsion of an implant?

WHAT HAPPENS IF:

I have menstrual cycle changes? This is a normal part of using Norplant; if the changes really bother you, taking a few cycles of combined pills or a medicine like ibuprofen may help (ask your clinician).

I don't get my period? This is normal in Norplant users. You are almost certainly not pregnant. However, if you don't get your period after having them regularly, you could be pregnant. You need to get tested for pregnancy if you have signs of pregnancy. If you are still worried about not getting periods, a cycle of combined pills may help.

I have spotting/breakthrough bleeding? This is normal and not harmful. If it is bothersome to you, a few cycles of low-dose combined pills and/or a pain reliever like ibuprofen might help. It is a good idea for your clinician to make sure you do not have an ectopic pregnancy or infection (including pelvic inflammatory disease).

I have heavy bleeding? If bothersome to you, a few cycles of low-dose combined pills, OR a medicine such as ibuprofen might help. Blood work may be done to make sure you are not anemic.

I have abdominal pain? If you have an ectopic pregnancy, you need to be treated. If you have ovarian cyst(s), implants can stay in place because these cysts usually go away on their own without surgery. Go back to clinic in 3 weeks to be sure that cysts are going away. If pain is from another cause, you need to be evaluated.

I have pain after insertion? Make sure bandaging is not too tight. Apply icepacks for 24 hours. Do not press on the implants for several days. Never press on the implants if they are tender. Take aspirin or a pain reliever such as ibuprofen.

If the site gets infected?
- *No abscess (itchy, red):* Implants usually do not need to be taken out. The area needs to be cleaned with an antiseptic and your clinician may have you take antibiotics. Go back to the clinic in 7 days.
- *Abscess (swollen, pus):* You need to take antibiotics and have the abscess drained. The implants will probably be taken out.

My breasts are tender? Some drugs that help are vitamin E, bromocriptine, tamoxifen or Danazol. A looser bra and taking a pain reliever such as ibuprofen may also help relieve tenderness. Ask your clinician what will best help you.

I get severe headaches? If you have severe headaches with blurred vision, flashing lights, temporary loss of vision, seeing zigzag lines, or have trouble speaking or moving, go to your clinician right away. Your clinician may need to remove the implants immediately.

I get headaches but they do not involve neurological symptoms? Treatment varies from person to person; sometimes implants have to be taken out, but often not.

I gain weight? Usually Norplant is not the cause of weight gain.

I have an allergic reaction? Rare; implants need to be taken out.

I lose hair? You may need to have implants taken out.

I have acne or skin changes? You may need to have implants taken out.

WHAT HAPPENS DURING REMOVAL OF NORPLANT?

- You can have the implants taken out at any time for any reason. Call 1-800-760-9030 for the name and phone number of a trained clinician near you who will take them out

- When you get the implants taken out, you clinician will numb the area like she or he did when you had the implants put in

- A small cut is made and a tool that grasps each implant from the side is used to take each one out (see picture to right)

- You should not be able to feel anything except for slight pulling or tugging. Tell your clinician if you feel any pain or discomfort during the procedure and he or she will make the area more numb

- Ask your clinician to show you the implants so that you see all six were removed

- If you feel tingling in your fingers, tell your clinician right away. It could mean that the implants were put in too deeply and removal may cause damage to your nerve (very rare)

- After all of the implants are taken out, a sticky bandage will hold the small cut together and another bandage will put pressure on the area to help it heal

- If you want to continue using Norplant, your clinician can put a new set in at the same time using the same small cut or new implants may be inserted in the other arm

- A medicine such as ibuprofen can help relieve pain you might have after removal

- After removal, other contraception should be used right away if you don't want to get pregnant

WHAT IF I WANT TO GET PREGNANT AFTER USING NORPLANT?

- After removal, fertility returns almost immediately
- Hormones disappear from the body within a week

If you have any questions, ask us at…
www.managingcontraception.com

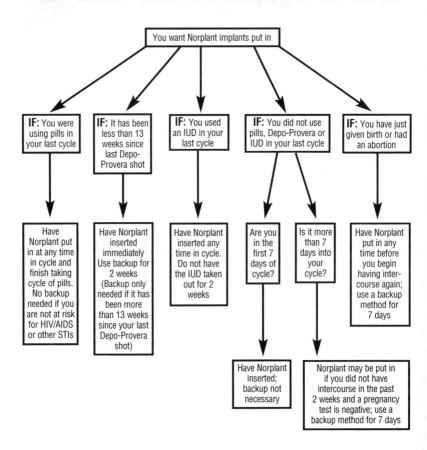

You want Norplant implants put in

IF: You were using pills in your last cycle

IF: It has been less than 13 weeks since last Depo-Provera shot

IF: You used an IUD in your last cycle

IF: You did not use pills, Depo-Provera or IUD in your last cycle

IF: You have just given birth or had an abortion

Have Norplant put in at any time in cycle and finish taking cycle of pills. No backup needed if you are not at risk for HIV/AIDS or other STIs

Have Norplant inserted immediately Use backup for 2 weeks (Backup only needed if it has been more than 13 weeks since your last Depo-Provera shot)

Have Norplant inserted any time in cycle. Do not have the IUD taken out for 2 weeks

Are you in the first 7 days of cycle?

Is it more than 7 days into your cycle?

Have Norplant put in any time before you begin having inter-course again; use a backup method for 7 days

Have Norplant inserted; backup not necessary

Norplant may be put in if you did not have intercourse in the past 2 weeks and a pregnancy test is negative; use a backup method for 7 days

NOTE: Norplant only protects against pregnancy. It does not protect against sexually transmitted infections. Therefore, you always need to use a condom if you are at risk of infection.

Adapted directly from the Manual of Medical Standards and Guidelines Planned Parenthood Federation of America July, 1998; Section III-B-1, Page 4

Contraceptive Implants: Implanon

WHAT IS IMPLANON?

- Single implant (slightly longer than one Norplant implant) put under the skin
- Contains the hormone, **etonogestrel**, that is released slowly each day
- Stays highly effective for 2-3 years

HOW EFFECTIVE IS IMPLANON?

Perfect use failure rate in first year: **0.05%**

Similar to Norplant: 1 out of every 2,000 women will become pregnant in the first year of use

Typical use failure rate in first year: **0.05%**

HOW DOES IMPLANON WORK?

- Within 24 hours of insertion, thick cervical mucus stops sperm from going through the cervix
- Stops ovulation
- Causes the lining of the uterus to stay thin

HOW MUCH DOES IMPLANON COST? Unknown; not yet available in the USA.

WHAT ARE THE ADVANTAGES OF IMPLANON?

- Implantation is more simple than for Norplant
- Very effective. Single decision and procedure may lead to long-term contraception
- In clinical trials many people choose to keep using Implanon
- Reduced risk of ectopic pregnancy
- Cramping or pain during periods or at the time of ovulation may get less
- All types of headaches may get better
- Low dose of progestin and no estrogen – dose is slightly higher than Norplant, but less than Depo-Provera
- May be used by some women who cannot take estrogen
- May lead to no periods which some women see as an advantage

WHAT ARE THE DISADVANTAGES OF IMPLANON?

- Does not protect against sexually transmitted infections, including HIV/AIDS
- Removal requires clinic visit, but is rarely difficult
- Irregular bleeding may lead to no periods in 22% of users which some women see as a disadvantage
- Headaches are the most common side effect
- Strongly suspect pregnancy if missed period comes after a series of regular cycles
- Discontinuation (the percentage of women who stopped using Norplant) ranged from 2% to 23% in 2 major studies. In both, the rates of amenorrhea (no periods) and prolonged bleeding were the same but the discontinuation rates varied widely

WHAT ARE THE RISKS OF IMPLANON? (see Norplant)

- Similar to Norplant (see page 137)
- Problems during removal happen much less often than with Norplant

WHO CAN USE IMPLANON?

- Similar to women who can use Norplant (see page 138)

HOW DO I START THE METHOD?

- See Norplant (page 140)

WHAT GUIDELINES DO I NEED TO FOLLOW?

- Irregular bleeding is normal. If your pattern of bleeding is unacceptable, go back to your clinician because there are some things that may be done to make your bleeding better
- You may not get periods. This is more common in Depo-Provera users and less common in Norplant users, as compared to possible Implanon users

WHAT HAPPENS IF:

- See Norplant (page 139) for how to manage possible side effects

WHAT IF I WANT TO GET PREGNANT AFTER USING IMPLANON?

- After removal, fertility returns almost immediately

WHAT IS FEMALE STERILIZATION?
(Tubal ligation or "getting your tubes tied"—permanent female contraception)

Surgery that blocks the fallopian tubes to prevent pregnancy—called tubal ligation or tubal sterilization. In 1995, 24% of married women said they have had a tubal ligation and 15% said that their husbands have had male sterilization—called vasectomy (see chapter 33, page 153). *[Chandra, 1998]* About half of female sterilizations in the USA are done right after a woman gives birth (within 48 hours of delivery). *[Peterson, 1998]*

HOW EFFECTIVE IS TUBAL LIGATION?

Failure rates differ by sterilization method and woman's age.

Failure rates for female sterilization methods *after 10 years* of use (each method explained below)

Method	Highest Failure rate
Tubal ligation after birth	0.8%
Silastic bands	1.8%
Partial tubal ligation	2.0%
Bipolar cautery	2.5%
Spring clip	3.7%

*U.S. Collaborative Review of Sterilization. The risk of pregnancy after tubal sterilization. Am J Obstet Gynecol 1996;174:1161-70.

- The above rates may differ from rates in private offices or clinics
- Younger women have higher failure rates because they have more remaining cycles
- All techniques must be done by a trained clinician in order for them to be most effective
- The filshie clip method is not included in above table

HOW DOES TUBAL LIGATION WORK?

The fallopian tubes are blocked so that eggs cannot get through to be fertilized. It will not change your monthly periods

STERILIZATION USING LAPAROSCOPY:

One type of sterilization is called laproscopic sterilization. A woman usually has to stay in the hospital for a day surgery and general anesthesia (being put to sleep) is usually recommended. During a laparoscopy, a tube with a viewing lens is inserted through the abdomen. The surgeon finds the fallopian tubes through this lens and then inserts another instrument through the same incision or a second one. The second instrument is used to close the fallopian tubes in one of the following ways:

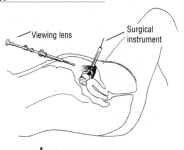

Laparoscopy

Diagrams of Techniques Using Laparoscopy

1. Bipolar cautery:
Both tubes are cauterized (burned) using an instrument that carries an electric current.

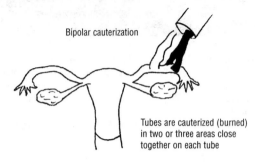

Bipolar cauterization

Tubes are cauterized (burned) in two or three areas close together on each tube

2. Hulka-Clemens clip:
A spring-loaded clip is placed on the tubes to block them. This method has high potential for being reversed if a woman chooses to try to regain fertility for a subsequent pregnancy.

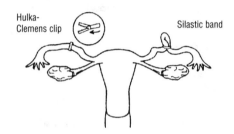

Hulka-Clemens clip

Silastic band

3. Silastic band:
A band is placed around the tubes to block them. This method may cause more pain after the procedure than other procedure.

Filshie clip

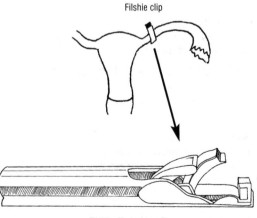

4. Filshie clip:
A hinge made of titanium with a curved silicone rubber clip is placed on the tubes to block them. This method, like the Hulka-Clemens clip, has better results if it needs to be reversed.

Filshie clip (enlarged)

METHODS OF TUBAL LIGATION AFTER A WOMAN GIVES BIRTH

During these procedures, local or general anesthesia is used and a woman can have the procedure done after she has given birth. A small incision is made in the lower abdomen or belly button so that the surgeon can see the fallopian tubes. The tubes are then closed ("ligated") using one of the following methods:

Pomeroy:
- Tubes are tied with a suture and then the tied-off loop is removed by cutting it out

Parkland/Pritchard:
- Tubes are tied in two places and then the portion in between is removed

Irving:
- Tubes are tied in two places and the portion in between is removed. The end of the tube connected to the uterus is then buried in the uterine wall

Uchida:
- Tubes are injected with saline solution. Muscular parts of tubes are divided and removed. The end of each tube is connected to the uterus and then buried in uterine wall

Kroener:
- The ends of the fallopian tubes (the fingerlike structures called fimbriae) are removed, which blocks the ends of the tubes

Techniques of Sterilization Afterbirth

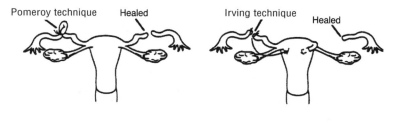

Pomeroy technique   Healed

Irving technique   Healed

Pritchard (Parkland) technique

Uchida technique

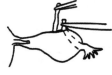

Kroener technique

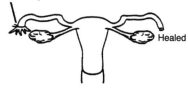

Healed

HOW MUCH DOES TUBAL LIGATION COST?

Managed-Care Setting	Public Provider Setting
$2500	$1200

WHAT ARE THE ADVANTAGES OF TUBAL LIGATION?

Menstrual: None

Sexual/psychological:
- May enjoy sex more because less fear of pregnancy

Cancers, tumors, and masses:
- May help protect against ovarian cancer

Other:
- Permanent
- Effective
- Requires only outpatient surgery (you do not have to stay in the hospital)

WHAT ARE THE DISADVANTAGES OF TUBAL LIGATION?

Menstrual:
- Possible changes in menstrual cycle (unlikely)
- None of the potential benefits of hormonal contraceptives

Sexual/psychological: Regret may occur (see page 139)

Cancers, tumors, and masses: None

Other:
- High cost up front
- If failure occurs, higher risk of ectopic pregnancy (10%-65% higher risk)
- Does not protect against sexually transmitted infections, including HIV/AIDS
- Not easily reversible. Most insurance companies will not pay for reversal

WHAT ARE THE RISKS OF TUBAL LIGATION? *[Peterson, 1997]*

	Minilaparotomy (smaller incision)	Laparoscopy
Minor problems	11.6% risk	6.0% risk
Major problems	1.5% risk	0.9% risk

- Minor problems may include infection or problems with the incision healing
- Major problems may include need for major surgery, due to hemorrhage (severe bleeding), or significant injuries to internal organs
- Major damage to blood vessels with laparoscopy occurs in 3-9 out of 10,000 procedures
- Death occurs in 1-2 out of 100,000 procedures (leading cause is from general anesthesia)

WHAT ARE THE LONG-TERM RISKS OF TUBAL LIGATION?

- Possible, although unlikely, risk of menstrual problems
- Regret (0.9%-26.0%). You are more likely to regret sterilization if you are young, have changed partners, have just given birth, have had a miscarriage or abortion, or have used public money for the procedure

WHO CAN USE TUBAL LIGATION?

Women who:
- Are certain they want no more children
- Are over age 21 (if using federal or state funds for sterilization)
- Have a medical condition that makes pregnancy dangerous
- Can safely have surgery

What About Adolescents? Not the best method, because women who are young usually have more regret and higher failure rates.

BEFORE YOU CHOOSE STERILIZATION, ASK YOURSELF THESE QUESTIONS:

Following are important questions to help you evaluate whether sterilization is right for you. If you answer "yes" to any question, talk to your clinician to figure out the best solution for you

☐ Have I considered other contraceptive options, including vasectomy for my partner? (If you are unsure, wait)

☐ Have I thought of all the reasons for choosing sterilization? (If you are unsure, wait)

☐ Is it possible that I will regret the decision? (If you are not sure, wait)

☐ Do I have questions about the details of the procedure including the anesthesia (being put to sleep)?

☐ Do I think that I may want to have the sterilization reversed?

☐ Do I understand the possibility of failure and risk of ectopic pregnancy?

☐ Do I understand how tubal ligation will affect my body?

☐ Do I understand that I will need to use condoms when at risk for sexually transmitted infections?

☐ Do I understand that I will need to return for regular Pap smears?

☐ Have all my questions been answered?

☐ Do I understand the informed consent papers?

Adapted from ACOG Technical Bulletin, April 1996.

HOW DO I START THE METHOD?

- You will need to give informed consent. It is a very good idea to involve your spouse or partner in the decision and the office visit when you formally consent to the procedure
- You can get a tubal sterilization any time in your cycle if you are certain you are not pregnant

WHAT HAPPENS AFTER THE PROCEDURE?

You will need to go back to the clinic or office within 2 weeks so that your clinician can check the site for any problems

FERTILITY AFTER USE

- You (and your partner) must assume that this is a permanent method
- Reversal is very expensive (most insurance companies will not pay for it) and success depends on the method that is used for sterilization, the age of the woman and the surgeon's ability to do microsurgery. Not all women can have sterilization reversed. Reversal success ranges from 60%-80%

You are in your early 20s and want tubal sterilization after you have had 2-3 children

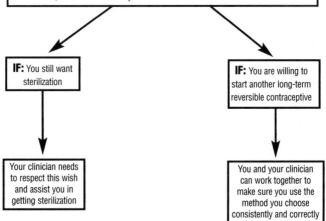

Your risk of regret after tubal sterilization is higher in the United States if you are:
- Young
- Unmarried (single, separated or divorced)
- Unmarried at the time of sterilization but married later, especially if your new husband wants a child with you
- Married now but become divorced later on
- On Medicaid or very poor
- African-American or Hispanic
- Have just given birth, had an abortion or miscarriage
- Thinking that sterilization is easy to reverse (it is not—it is expensive and only 60 - 80% effective)

You have some other options:
- You may want to wait until your later 20s or early 30s for sterilization
- You may want to use effective long-term contraception: Copper T 380-A IUD, or Norplant, or Depo-Provera
- In the end, the final decision is yours to make

IF: You still want sterilization

IF: You are willing to start another long-term reversible contraceptive

Your clinician needs to respect this wish and assist you in getting sterilization

You and your clinician can work together to make sure you use the method you choose consistently and correctly

WHAT IS MALE STERILIZATION (VASECTOMY)?

Permanent male contraception. Performed in a minor surgical procedure in an office or clinic that involves cutting and tying off or cauterizing (burning) the vas deferens—the tubes that transport sperm out of the scrotum (sac) from the testicles. A no-scalpel method allows the surgeon to go through the scrotum and perform the sterilization with a special instrument that gently punctures the skin. Local anesthesia is used and vasectomy takes about half an hour to complete.

HOW EFFECTIVE IS VASECTOMY?

Perfect-use failure rate in first year: 0.10%
Typical-use failure rate in first year: Unknown *[Trussell J, Contraceptive Technology, 1998]*
• Vasectomy is potentially the most effective of all contraceptive methods because men can have their ejaculate checked for sperm periodically—for example, 1, 2, or 5 years after the procedure as well as immediately after the procedure

HOW DOES VASECTOMY WORK?

Blocked vas deferens prevent sperm from moving into seminal fluid and being ejaculated. (NOTE: A man is still able to ejaculate fluid during an orgasm, but no sperm comes out in the ejaculate. Orgasms feel the same to men after vasectomy.)

HOW MUCH DOES VASECTOMY COST?

	Managed-Care Setting	*Public Provider Setting*
	$755.70	$353.28 *[Trussell, 1995; Smith, 1993]*

WHAT ARE THE ADVANTAGES OF VASECTOMY?

Sexual/psychological:
• Sexual intercourse may be more enjoyable because less fear of pregnancy
• Man can take on an important role in contraception
• Nothing to interrupt sex
• Woman does not have to worry about contraception
• No supplies or further clinic visits needed after sperm count has been shown to be zero

Cancers, tumors, and masses: None
Other:
• More simple, safe and effective than female sterilization
• Cost-effective (cheaper than female sterilization)
• General anesthesia is not necessary (as it is in female sterilization), which reduces the risk of serious complications
• Very effective
• Permanent
• Procedure can be done quickly

WHAT ARE THE DISADVANTAGES OF VASECTOMY?

Sexual/ psychological:
• Man may regret later
• Need to use a backup method the first 20 times a man ejaculates

Cancers, tumors, and masses:
• Very slight association with increased risk of prostate cancer (may be caused by other factors, though) *[Goldstein, 1997]*

153

Other:
- Does not protect against sexually transmitted infections, including HIV/AIDS
- Short-term discomfort, bruising, swelling
- Initial high cost
- Needs surgical procedure
- Needs trained clinician, technical assistance, medicines, sterile conditions

WHAT ARE THE RISKS OF VASECTOMY?
- No-scalpel method (29% of vasectomies in the U.S.) has less problems
- Uncommonly, bleeding or infection at or near incision site
- Blood clots in scrotum

WHO CAN USE VASECTOMY?
Males of any age who:
- Want a permanent, effective method of contraception
- Have partners who should not get pregnant for health reasons
- Have no infections on the skin or scrotum at present time
- Have no genital tract infection (such as gonorrhea, syphilis, chlamydia)
- Have no general infection (such as the flu)

What About Adolescents? Not the best method because young people tend to have more regret.

HOW DO I START THE METHOD?
- You will need to have a general physical exam and go over your medical history with your clinician
- You will need to give informed consent
- Understand that the method is permanent
- Before the surgery you will need to wash the genital area and upper thighs; wear clean, loose-fitting clothes to clinic; do not take any medicines 24 hours before the vasectomy unless you and your clinician agree on a different plan

Vasectomy Procedure

1. Clinician finds vas deferens.
2. A very small incision is made.

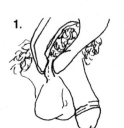
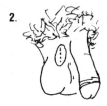
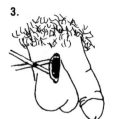
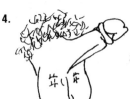

3. Vas deferens is lifted out, cut, tied and often cauterized (burned).

4. Small incisions are stitched and man can walk out of office.

WHAT GUIDELINES DO I NEED TO FOLLOW?

- Abstain from sex or use backup contraception the next 20 times you ejaculate or for 3 months
- Return to clinic with semen sample at that time
- **Do not consider vasectomy effective until it is confirmed that no sperm are present**
- If possible, ice scrotum for 4 hours to make swelling go down
- Rest for 2 days after the procedure
- Keep incision clean and dry; do not soak in water (baths, jacuzzi)
- Wear snug underwear and pants (decreases swelling and gives support)
- You may have sexual intercourse 2-3 days after, but use a backup method
- Return to clinic within 7 days to remove stitches, if necessary
- Return if your partner misses her period and thinks she is pregnant
- Return immediately if you have a high fever above 100°F, bleeding and/or pus from incision site, pain, heat, swelling or redness at site

DO I NEED TO CONSULT MY CLINICIAN? ASK YOURSELF:

Following are important questions to help you evaluate whether vasectomy is working well for you. If you answer "yes" to any question, talk to your clinician to figure out the best solution for you

☐ Were there sperm under the microscope when my semen was tested?
☐ Do I have any signs of infection (bleeding, redness, pain, or pus at the site)?

WHAT HAPPENS IF:

The site gets infected? It may be treated with antibiotics. Any abscesses (pus-filled swollen areas) need to be drained and treated.

I have bruising? Apply warm, moist packs to scrotum. Provide scrotal support (snug fitting underwear or pants). Usually it will go away on its own.

I have pain at the site? If no infection, provide support for the scrotum (snug fitting underwear or pants) and take pain relievers as needed.

I have severe swelling? If large and painful, you may need surgery. Provide scrotal support if infection or bruising.

WHAT IF I AND MY PARTNER WANT TO GET PREGNANT AFTER VASECTOMY?

- Man (and partner) must understand that vasectomy is a permanent procedure
- Reversal using microsurgery techniques now result in pregnancy rates of 50% or higher and sperm returns to ejaculate in over 90% of men
- All of these factors can affect success of reversal:
  - *skill of microsurgeon*
  - *length of time from vasectomy*
  - *presence of antibodies that attack sperm*
  - *partner's fertility*
  - *method used for vasectomy*

Researchers continue to work on developing new contraceptive methods. Although it will take a while until some of these methods are available in the U.S., others are close to being approved and put on the market. This chapter presents up-to-date information on these exciting new developments.

VAGINAL HORMONAL METHODS: rings, suppositories & microbicides

Methods that are inserted into the vagina are being developed. Some of them include:

- An estrogen-progestin vaginal ring (will be called NuvaRing) that is left in for 3 weeks and taken out in the fourth week of the cycle. NuvaRing is a soft, flexible ring made of a material called ethylene vinylacetate (EVA). It is about 5.4 centimeters in diameter and about 4 millimeters in thickness. It contains the estrogen, **ethynil estradiol,** and the progesterone, **etonogestrel,** which are released into the body through the ring. A woman inserts the ring into her vagina at the beginning of her cycle where it stays for 3 weeks. After 3 weeks, she removes it and 1 week later she inserts a new ring. Most women experience a menstrual-like period during the week they are not using the ring. The ring prevents **NuvaRing (vaginal ring)** pregnancy in the following ways: estrogen and progesterone stop ovulation and thicken cervical mucus, making it difficult for sperm to get through the cervix. Data on effectiveness are still being collected from clinical trials. It is anticipated that the effectiveness of NuvaRing will be similar to combined oral contraceptive pills when used correctly. Side effects are similar to those of combined pills.

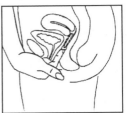

- Progestin-only vaginal rings that are worn continuously
- Progesterone suppositories put into the vagina once a day
- Vaginal hormonal pills placed in the vagina. Ethinyl estradiol (50 micrograms) and levonorgestrel (250 micrograms) for 21 days, then 7 days off. Marketed as Lovelle in Brazil since 1999. Main reason to use: nausea or vomiting when taking pills by mouth. This is the same dosage of hormones in the combined pill Ovral
- Effective vaginal microbicides (that kill bacteria), and are also spermicidal (kill sperm), will probably NOT be available for at least 10 years

PROGESTIN-ONLY IMPLANTS

Some new implant contraceptives are being developed that contain only a progestin. The table below shows the information that is known about the number of implants, the type of progestin, and how long the implants are effective.

NAME	# IMPLANTS	HORMONE	LENGTH OF USE
Norplant 2	2	levonorgestrel	3 years
Implanon	1	etonogestrel	3 years
Uniplant	1	nomegestrol	1 year
Nestorone	1	nestorone	2 years
Annuelle	pellets	norethindrone	unavailable

METHODS APPLIED TO THE SKIN

- Estrogen/progestin patches worn on the skin and absorbed into the body. A contraceptive "patch" is currently being tested by researchers in the U.S.
- Hormonal gels that are put on the skin

INTRAUTERINE DEVICES

- Gynefix Copper IUD has a "frameless" design and does not take a lot of space in the uterus. This IUD has a low expulsion rate and many people continue to use it after one year (90%). The failure rate after 3 years is 0.5% *[Grimes, 1998]*

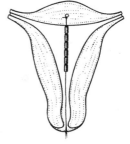

Gynefix intrauterine copper implant

FEMALE BARRIERS

- New types of female condoms
- Lea's shield: "one size fits all" silicone rubber diaphragm
- Femcap: silicone rubber cervical cap in 3 sizes
- Protectaid: new vaginal sponges
- Microbicides which are also spermicidal (kill bacteria and sperm)

MALE METHODS

In the past, contraception has been mostly a woman's responsibility. Now, a big question on the minds of many people is, "What methods are being developed for men?" Right now, men have the options of condoms, withdrawal, and vasectomy, whereas women have many methods from which to choose. Here is the latest information on what methods are in the works for men:

- Male hormonal methods under development often use the hormones progestin or gonadotropin-releasing hormone (GnRH) to suppress other hormones (FSH and LH) which then decrease sperm and testosterone production. Both injectables and implants are being developed
- Immunocontraception: These methods stop the reproductive process through an immune system reaction
- "Temporary sterilization"—a clinician injects the vas deferens with a substance that blocks sperm
- Anti-sperm drugs: Gossypol, a substance taken from cottonseed oil, was developed to kill sperm. Another anti-sperm substance called Triptolide is being developed

Can We Protect Ourselves AND Still Have Fun?

Yes! To prove it, here are 99 sexual things you can do while staying infection-free:

1. Erotic massage
2. Stroke each other's hair
3. Shower together
4. Hold hands
5. Play footsie
6. Light candles
7. Long hugs
8. Have phone sex
9. Watch erotic videos
10. Mutual masturbation
11. Fantasize
12. Read erotic stories
13. Write your own erotic stories
14. Tell each other your fantasies
15. Foot massage
16. Cuddle
17. Sleep in bed together
18. Go out for a romantic dinner
19. Look at erotic magazines
20. Strip for your partner
21. Go to a strip club together
22. French kiss
23. Feed each other
24. Hand massage
25. Gaze into each other's eyes
26. Play dress-up
27. Take erotic photographs
28. Flatter each other
29. Body painting
30. Body painting...with food
31. Draw or paint each other
32. Kiss each other's necks
33. Nibble each other's ears
34. Whisper in each other's ears
35. Kiss in public
36. Watch a sexy movie at home
37. Take a bubble bath
38. Relax in a jacuzzi
39. Go skinny dipping
40. Take a moonlight walk
41. Cook dinner together
42. Cuddle by the fireplace
43. Give your partner flowers
44. Tickle each other
45. Tie up your partner
46. Talk dirty to each other
47. Role play
48. Flirt with each other
49. Pretend you just met
50. Use a vibrator
51. Wear sexy lingerie
52. Aromatherapy
53. Eat chocolate together
54. Write love letters
55. Have e-sex
56. Relax on a beach together
57. Look up sexy Internet sites
58. Go on a vacation together
59. Tickle each other with feathers
60. Cross-dress
61. Go to an adult toy store
62. Sleep side-by-side ("spooning")
63. Use a dildo
64. Shop together for sexy lingerie
65. Go dancing together
66. Write poems for each other
67. Wear perfume or cologne
68. Dress up and go to a formal event
69. Watch a sexy movie in the theater
70. Kiss each other's stomachs
71. Spank you partner
72. Listen to erotic music
73. Look at stars on a clear night
74. Make out in a library
75. Dance naked together at home
76. Send each other a romantic gift
78. Make your own erotic movie
79. Lay on the grass and look at clouds
80. Have breakfast in bed
81. Give each other romantic gifts
82. Go camping in a remote location
83. Write each other little love notes
84. Go on a picnic
85. Butterfly kisses (with your eyelashes)
86. Work with clay together
87. "Dry" humping
88. Go on a date
89. Burn incense
90. Feed each other
91. Play doctor
92. Wrestle with each other
93. Walk in the woods
94. Watch your lover sleep
95. Pick wildflowers
96. Be a voyeur
97. Look at erotic art
98. Serenade your lover
99. **Let your mind go... the possibilities are infinite!**

NOTE: In order to stay infection-free, you must avoid contact with or exchange of another person's body fluids—specifically, blood, vaginal fluids, semen, preejaculatory fluid ("precum"), and breast milk. Some infections can also be spread when infected skin touches uninfected skin. All of the above activities are considered safe as long as contact with body fluids and infected skin is not involved.

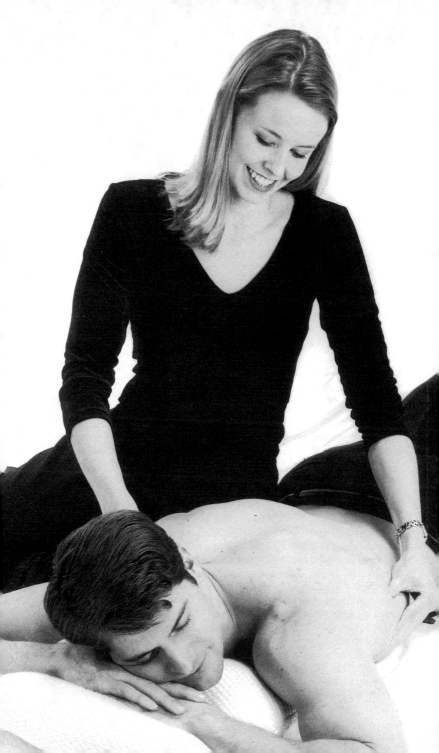

C H A P T E R   3 5

Sexually Transmitted Infections (STIs)
www.ashastd.org

Since women and men who use contraceptives are also at risk for sexually transmitted infections (STIs), we have included in this book information on the most important infections. NOTE: The terms "STI" and "STD" mean the same thing. The authors prefer the term "infection" to "disease" (as in sexually transmitted disease, or STD) because "infection" has less negative connotations associated with it than "disease."

Information in this chapter has been adapted from the *1998 Guidelines for Sexually Transmitted Diseases* published by the Centers for Disease Control and Prevention *[CDC, 1998]*. The specific treatment and prevention methods presented below are from that document.

WHAT DO I NEED TO DO TO PREVENT GETTING OR PASSING AN INFECTION?

Preventing the spread of STIs requires that people who are at risk for transmitting or acquiring infections change their behaviors. The first step in prevention is identifying any behaviors (past or current) that may put you at risk for infection. It is a good idea to discuss any possible risks with a health care provider, who can help you decide on the appropriate actions to take.

The most effective way to prevent sexual transmission of infections is to avoid sexual intercourse with an infected partner—abstinence (see chapter 14, page 37). It is important to note that certain infections may be transmitted through other sexual behaviors. For example, it is possible to spread herpes orally (through kissing or oral sex). Using condoms or dental dams (square pieces of latex) during oral sex may help prevent the spread of some of these infections. Both partners should get tested for STIs, including HIV, before having sexual intercourse. If you choose to have sexual intercourse with a partner whose infection status is unknown or who is infected with HIV or another STI, a new condom should be used for each act of intercourse.

Telling your sex partner(s) that you have a sexually transmitted infection can be very difficult to do but it is one of the most important things you can do. Being honest with past and present partners (if they are at risk of infection) will help them get treatment if they are infected and will help stop the spread of the infection to other people.

Prevention Methods

Male Condoms:

- Used consistently and correctly, condoms are effective in preventing many infections, including HIV
- Condoms are more likely to fail from incorrect or inconsistent use, rather than from breaking during intercourse

Female Condoms:

- Laboratory studies indicate that the female condom (Reality) is an effective barrier to viruses, including HIV
- Used consistently, the female condom should substantially reduce risk for STIs

Condoms and Spermicides:

- Whether condoms used with vaginal spermicides are more effective than condoms used without vaginal spermicides is unknown
- Thus, regular use of condoms, with or without spermicide or vaginal spermicides, is recommended

Vaginal Spermicides, Sponges, and Diaphragms:

- Vaginal spermicides used alone without condoms help reduce the risk for gonorrhea and chlamydia
- **Vaginal spermicides do not protect against HIV infection**
- Diaphragm use has been shown to give some protection against cervical gonorrhea, chlamydia, and trichomoniasis ("trich")
- Do not assume that vaginal sponges or diaphragms protect women against HIV infection

Hormonal Contraception, Surgical Sterilization, and Hysterectomy (removal of uterus):

- Women who are not at risk of pregnancy might incorrectly perceive themselves to be at no risk for STIs, including HIV infection. Non-barrier contraceptive methods offer no protection against HIV or other STIs.
- Hormonal contraceptives (pills, Norplant, and Depo-Provera) have been associated in some research with increased cervical infection and increased HIV infection. BUT, research is inconsistent, so we do not know for sure
- Women who use hormonal or intrauterine contraception, have been surgically sterilized, or have had their uteruses removed need to use condoms if they are at risk for infection (e.g., new partner, multiple partners, or have a partner who has had multiple partners)

Vaccines:

- One of the best ways to prevent sexually transmitted infections is through immunization, or giving people vaccines before they have been exposed. The only vaccines that are available currently are for hepatitis A and hepatitis B. It is a very good idea to get vaccinated against these infections—ask your clinician. Vaccines are being developed for other infections, including herpes and HIV, but it will be a while until these vaccines are available to the public. In the meantime, protecting yourself by abstaining from sexual activity that puts you at risk (anal, oral, and vaginal intercourse) is the best way to prevent infection. Using condoms *correctly every time* you have sex is the next best way to protect yourself and your partner(s)

Drug and Alcohol Use and Infections:
- Using drugs or alcohol may increase the likelihood of not using a method of protection, or not using a method consistently and correctly. It is important to know that being drunk or high may, therefore, increase your risk of getting a sexually transmitted infection. If you use injection drugs (e.g., heroine, cocaine), you may be at risk of getting or passing HIV. It is important that you enroll or continue in a drug-treatment program. Do not, under any circumstances, use injection equipment (e.g., needles and syringes) that has been used by another person. If needles can be obtained legally in the community, obtain clean needles. If you continue to use injection equipment that has been used by other people, you should first clean the equipment with bleach and water. (Disinfecting with bleach does not sterilize the equipment and does not guarantee that HIV is inactivated. However, for injecting-drug users, thoroughly and consistently cleaning injection equipment with bleach should reduce the rate of HIV transmission when equipment is shared.)

INFECTIONS IN SPECIAL POPULATIONS

Pregnant Women
It is recommended that you get tested for these infections:
- *Syphilis:* all pregnant women need to be tested at their first visit to a clinician
- *Hepatitis B:* all pregnant women need to be tested at their first visit
- *Gonorrhea:* women who are at risk or living in an area where rates of gonorrhea are high need to be tested at their first visit
- *Chlamydia:* women at increased risk (women under 25 years old, women who have a new sex partner or more than one sex partner, women whose partners have other partners) need to be tested in their third trimester
- *HIV screening test:* offered to all pregnant women at their first prenatal visit
- *Bacterial vaginosis (BV):* Women who have bacterial vaginosis may be at high risk for preterm (early) labor and need to be tested early in the second trimester
- *Papanicolaou (Pap) smear (test for effects of papilloma virus infection and screens for cervical cancer):* If no Pap smear has been done in the past year, a woman needs to have a pap at the first visit

Other Concerns:
- Pregnant women who have genital herpes infection, Hepatitis B infection, primary cytomegalovirus (CMV) infection, or Group B streptococcal infection and women who have syphilis and are allergic to penicillin may require expert consultation or care during pregnancy and birth
- If there are no herpes sores during the third trimester, a routine test for herpes simplex virus (HSV) is not needed for women who have recurrent genital herpes. However, testing these women at the time of delivery may be useful in guiding treatment of the baby. Cesarean section is not recommended for women who do not have sores at the time of delivery
- The presence of genital warts is not a reason for cesarean section

Adolescents
- With a few exceptions, all U.S. teens can consent without parental involvement to the confidential testing, diagnosis and treatment of sexually transmitted infections (see table on page 18)
- Medical care for infections can be given to adolescents even if parents do not give their consent
- Clinicians know that confidentiality is very important to adolescents

HIV/AIDS is complex, inconsistent in its presentation and, above all, deeply concerning to people who are infected and partners and individuals trying to avoid infection. The following is just a brief overview. For more information, contact the Centers for Disease Control AIDS Hotline: (800) 342-2437.

What causes HIV?

- The Human Immunodeficiency Virus (HIV) is the virus that causes AIDS (Acquired Immunodeficiency Syndrome)
- HIV is passed through certain human body fluids (blood, semen, vaginal fluids, and breast milk)
- HIV can also be passed from mother to child during pregnancy and delivery
- HIV is NOT passed through casual contacts like hugging or holding hands, sharing eating utensils or toilet seats, or kissing (unless both partners have open sores in their mouths)
- **Anyone can get HIV if they engage in a behavior where body fluids are exchanged (such as sharing needles during injection drug use, tattooing or piercing; having unprotected vaginal, oral, or anal intercourse; and breastfeeding a baby if you are HIV positive). It does not matter what gender, race, ethnicity, sexual orientation, or age you are. It is not who you are but what you do that puts you at risk of HIV infection**

What are the symptoms of HIV?

- HIV attacks the immune system, eventually making it unable to fight off other infections
- There are usually no symptoms early on. Many people have flu-like symptoms (fever, chills, and aches) but most people do not recognize they are infected unless they are tested (see below). In fact, it is estimated that about half of the people infected with HIV do not know it
- Later symptoms may include weight loss, fever, cough, rash, diarrhea, night sweats and swollen lymph nodes. Because the immune system is weak, it is possible to get other serious infections including cancer, pneumonia and tuberculosis (many of which lead to death)
- Once inside the body, HIV begins attacking the T-cells (an important part of the immune system) and the virus copies itself over and over again. Even if a person seems totally healthy, the virus can be copying itself and slowly making the immune system weak

How long will it take from the time of HIV infection to get AIDS?

- Ranges from several months to many years (average time is 10 years)
- Now there are more and more people infected with HIV who have not yet developed AIDS because of effective medicines (some have even been infected up to 20 years and are still relatively healthy)

How will I be tested for HIV?

- Blood tests are used to look for antibodies to the virus
- You must give informed consent in order to have an HIV test
- **IMPORTANT:** From the time of exposure, it can take up to 6 months for a person to have a positive HIV test. Therefore, if you have a negative test soon after exposure, or are exposed again, you need to get tested again in 6 months to be sure of your HIV status
- **Every person needs to be tested for HIV and re-tested if another risk has occurred— knowing your HIV status can help prevent the spread of the infection. Anonymous and free testing is available in many locations**

- To be diagnosed with AIDS, a person must have a positive HIV blood test and one of the following: an opportunistic infection (there are currently 26 that are associated with AIDS); a cancer (the most frequent is Kaposi's sarcoma); HIV wasting syndrome (severe weight loss); AIDS dementia complex (severe mental dysfunction); or a T-cell count below 200 (a healthy person has a T-cell count between 800 and 1,500)

How will I be treated for HIV?
- **There is NO CURE for HIV/AIDS.** Although AIDS eventually develops in almost all people who have HIV, there are currently many drugs available that help stop the virus from copying itself and stop the virus from further damaging the immune system. There are also drugs that prevent the development of opportunistic infections. These drugs have extended the lives of many people who have HIV. Therefore, it is critical that you seek medical care immediately if you are HIV-positive. Treatment is often dramatically effective and should be considered by all persons with HIV
- Side effects of these drugs can be severe and the drugs can be very expensive, depending on what type of health insurance you have (if any)
- For more information about HIV/AIDS treatments, contact the Centers for Disease Control AIDS Hotline (800) 342-2437

What about my sex partner(s)?
- It is extremely important that you tell all of your past and present sex partners if you are infected with HIV
- Telling sex partners, although it can be difficult, is the only thing that will stop them from spreading HIV to other people. Contact the AIDS Hotline (800) 342-2437 to ask for an organization in your area that can help you talk to your partner(s) or will do it anonymously for you

What if I am pregnant or want to get pregnant in the future?
- HIV can be passed from mother to child during pregnancy, birth, and breastfeeding
- All pregnant women should be offered HIV testing as soon as possible
- Drugs are currently available that make it much less likely that a mother will pass HIV to her baby while the baby is still in the uterus
- Tell your clinician if you are HIV-positive and pregnant. The sooner treatment begins, the less likely your baby is to be infected with HIV

STI's Which Tend to Cause Genital Ulcers (Sores)

CHANCROID (SHAN-kroyd)

What causes chancroid?
- A type of bacteria
- Infection is passed by coming into contact with an ulcer (sore) on another person

What are the symptoms of chancroid?
- Usually one or more painful ulcers in or around the genital area
- Men are more likely than women to have visible signs of infection

How will I be tested for chancroid?
- Your clinician will take a sample from the ulcer(s) and examine it under a microscope
- Infected people also need to be tested for herpes and syphilis (infections that also cause genital ulcers)

How will I be treated for chancroid?
- Antibiotics taken by mouth or given as an injection usually cure chancroid
- After treatment, you will need to be examined again in 3-7 days. If the sores have not gotten better, your clinician needs to check to see if you have another infection, including HIV, if you did not take your medicine as directed, or if the strain of bacteria might be resistant to the drugs you were given
- Time required for complete healing depends on the size of the sores. Large sores may take more than 2 weeks to heal
- It may take longer for men who have not been circumcised to heal if they have sores under the foreskin

What about my sex partner(s)?
- Any people with whom you have had sexual contact within 10 days since your symptoms started need to be examined and treated *even if* they do not have any symptoms

What if I am pregnant or want to get pregnant in the future?
- Some antibiotics cannot be used during pregnancy (e.g., ciprofoxacin)
- There have been no reports of chancroid causing problems in a developing baby
- Talk to your clinician about the best treatment for you and your baby

What causes herpes?

- Herpes Simplex Virus Type 1 (HSV-1) and Herpes Simplex Virus Type 2 (HSV-2) cause the infection
- Both strains of the virus can infect the mouth and the genitals (sores on the mouth are also called "cold sores" or "fever blisters")
- Herpes can be passed during vaginal-penile contact, oral-anal contact, and oral-genital contact (for example, you can get herpes on your genitals if someone who has a cold sore on their mouth performs oral sex on you)
- An infected mother can pass herpes to her baby in the womb or during birth
- Herpes can be passed to other places on the body by touching the sores (fingers, eyes, and other body areas). To prevent this, do not touch the area during an outbreak. If you do, wash your hands as soon as possible with soap and water to kill the herpes virus
- Babies (and adults) can get herpes if someone with a cold sore kisses them. Babies can not fight off infections as well as adults and might have serious problems if they get infected. Refrain from kissing if you have a cold sore
- *The virus can be spread **even if** you do not have active sores. In fact, you are most likely to spread the virus right before you get an outbreak of sores. During this time, you may feel tingling or itching in the area, called **prodromal** symptoms, which can warn you that an outbreak is coming*
- *The virus can also be spread **without any symptoms**. Therefore, you need to use a condom during sexual activity with new or uninfected sex partners and engage in honest dialogue about your infection since condoms are not completely effective in preventing transmission. You and your partner may also discuss the options of having unprotected sex and facing the risks that are involved*

What are the symptoms of herpes?

- Many people with herpes infection do not have any symptoms. It is possible to transmit the virus even if no symptoms (sores) are present (see above)
- Small, itchy, painful bumps in or around the genital area or on or around the mouth or lips. The bumps become blisters and may break, causing painful sores. The sores go away and may recur (some people gets sores once a month, some once every few years, and some never get sores again)
- Possibly swollen lymph nodes on the neck or in the pelvic area
- Possibly flu-like symptoms during the first outbreak (fever, chills, aches)

How will I be tested for herpes?

- Your clinician will take a sample from the sores and test it for the herpes virus
- The most specific test for herpes is conducted when you have sores. Your clinician will take a sample from the sore and lab results will tell you whether you have Type 1 or Type 2 infection
- In 1999, the FDA approved two new blood tests for herpes (Pockit® and Premier). Blood tests are often used when a person has concerns about herpes, but does not have any visible symptoms. These new tests will be able to identify the virus type, but not the place of infection (i.e., oral versus genital). Ask your clinician if you are interested in getting a herpes blood test

How will I be treated for herpes?

- **There is no cure for herpes.** Drugs (e.g., acyclovir, famciclovir, valacyclovir) are now available that you can take daily to help make outbreaks less likely to occur
- You can also take these drugs to prevent an outbreak or to make it less severe
- During outbreaks, soaking in Aveeno baths (available in drug stores), wearing loose-fitting clothing, and keeping the area clean and dry can help the healing process and help relieve pain
- Outbreaks are sometimes related to stress in your life. Learning to manage stress (eating right, exercise, getting enough sleep, relaxation) may help minimize outbreaks

What about my sex partner(s)?

- Any people with whom you have had recent sexual contact need to be examined and treated if they develop symptoms
- Do not engage in sexual activity when you have active sores or find safe alternatives that do not involve skin-to-skin contact

What if I am pregnant or want to get pregnant in the future?

- Herpes can be passed from mother to child. The risk is high (30%-50%) among women who get their first infection near the time of delivery. The risk is low (3%) among women who have a history of recurrent herpes and women who get herpes during the first half of pregnancy
- Women whose partners have oral or genital herpes and women who do not know if their partner is infected with herpes need to avoid unprotected oral and genital sex during late pregnancy
- Cesarean section (C-section) may be necessary if a woman has active herpes sores at the time of birth. Even C-section does not completely eliminate the risk of passing herpes to the baby
- Some infections are more dangerous during pregnancy than when a woman is not pregnant. Herpes is potentially very dangerous for a pregnant woman's baby. **CONDOMS MUST BE USED BY PREGNANT WOMEN AT THE RISK FOR HERPES, SYPHILIS, HPV, OR ANY SEXUALLY TRANSMITTED INFECTION.**

SYPHILIS (SIF-ih-lis)

What causes syphilis?
- A type of bacteria (*T. pallidum*)
- The bacteria need to be in mucus membranes to survive. It can be passed through oral, anal, and vaginal-penile intercourse
- An infected mother can pass syphilis to her unborn baby

What are the symptoms of syphilis?
- *Primary stage:* first sign is a *chancre* (pronounce *shayn-ker*), a red, pea-sized, painless ulcer in the area where the infection occurred (on the penis, vulva, or mouth)
- *Secondary stage:* red, itchy rash all over body, including the palms of hands and the soles of feet. This may not be noticed by all people because some may have fewer symptoms
- *Latent syphilis:* this is the time when a person tests positive for syphilis but has no symptoms (within 2-6 weeks after the symptoms of primary and secondary stage go away)
- *Tertiary syphilis (third stage):* if syphilis is not treated early on, it can lead to *severe* problems, including sores in the internal organs and eyes, heart disease, brain and spinal cord disorders, and brain damage leading to insanity

How will I be tested for syphilis?
- A laboratory test is used to look for syphilis antibodies
- More than one test needs to be done to get reliable results
- It is a good idea to get an HIV test if you have been infected with syphilis

How will I be treated for syphilis?
- You will get a shot of penicillin
- If you are allergic to penicillin, tell your clinician. Other antibiotics can be used
- After a shot of penicillin, watch for signs like headache and muscle pain, and return to the clinic if you get any of these reactions to treatment
- Latent and third-stage syphilis can also be treated with antibiotics (but you may need to stay in the hospital if the infection is severe)

What about my sex partner(s)?
- Syphilis can be passed only when a chancre is present (not usually after the first year of infection). But, anyone with whom you have had sexual contact should be tested for syphilis and treated if necessary

What if I am pregnant or want to get pregnant in the near future?
- An infected mother can pass syphilis to her unborn baby if she remains untreated
- Infection in unborn babies often causes brain damage
- It is a good idea to be screened in the first trimester of pregnancy for syphilis. If you are treated, your baby will not be at risk
- **It is very important for pregnant women at risk for becoming infected with syphilis to use condoms with every act of sexual intercourse**

STI's Which Tend to Cause Infections in the Urethra and Cervix

What causes nongonococcal urethritis (NGU)?
• An infection of the urethra caused by something other than gonorrhea. NGU means that after testing, gonorrhea has been ruled out as the cause of the infection. Other sexually transmitted organisms are usually the cause (e.g., chlamydia)

What are the symptoms of nongonococcal urethritis?
• *Men:* painful urination, frequent urination, or white or yellow discharge from the penis
• *Women:* likely to have no symptoms. If there are symptoms, they may include itching and burning during urination, or unusual discharge from the vagina

How will I be tested for nongonococcal urethritis?
• A laboratory test is used to look for the bacteria under a microscope
• Testing for chlamydia is strongly recommended. Very accurate tests are available and the symptoms of these infections are similar and may affect treatment

How will I be treated for nongonococcal urethritis?
• It is usually treated with antibiotics (e.g., azithromycin, doxycycline, erythromycin, or metronidazole) taken orally in a single dose or for 7-14 days
• Go back to your clinician if your symptoms do not go away
• Do not have sex until you have been tested and the infection is definitely gone (even after you finish the medicine)

What about my sex partner(s)?
• All people with whom you have had sexual contact in the past 60 days need to get tested and treated if they are infected

What if I am pregnant or want to get pregnant in the future?
• If you are pregnant and have any symptoms of infection, tell your clinician and you will be treated
• Some antibiotics cannot be used during pregnancy, but safe, effective treatments are available for virtually all women

CHLAMYDIA (kla-MIH-dee-a)

What causes chlamydia?
- A type of bacteria
- Chlamydia is the most common sexually transmitted infection in the U.S. It causes an estimated 4 million infections annually, primarily among sexually active adolescents and young adults
- Spread through vaginal, oral, and anal intercourse

What are the symptoms of chlamydia?
- *Women:* In early infection, *about 75% of women do not have any symptoms.* If there are symptoms they may include unusual discharge from the vagina, burning during urination, or unexplained vaginal bleeding between periods. In later infection they may include pain in lower abdomen, bleeding between periods, or low-grade fever
- *Men:* In early infection, *about 30-50% of men do not have any symptoms.* If there are symptoms they may include unusual discharge from the penis, burning during urination, itching and burning around the urethral opening, pain and swelling of the testicles, or low-grade fever (the last two symptoms may mean the man has *epididymitis*, an infection of the epididymis)
- If untreated, chlamydia can lead to serious problems for women (pelvic inflammatory disease (PID), ectopic pregnancy, and infertility). Without treatment, about 20-40% of women with chlamydia may develop PID

How will I be tested for chlamydia?
- Screening for chlamydia is available and strongly recommended if you are sexually active because you can have chlamydia without any symptoms
- A sample is taken using a cervical or penile swab
- A laboratory test is used to diagnose chlamydia

How will I be treated for chlamydia?
- Treated with antibiotics (e.g., azithromycin, doxycycline, erythromycin) taken orally in one dose or for 7-14 days
- People who have chlamydia are also likely to have gonorrhea so clinicians often treat for both infections
- You do not have to be retested for chlamydia after finishing treatment unless your symptoms do not go away or you have been exposed again

What about my sex partner(s)?
- All people with whom you have had sexual contact in the past 60 days need to get tested and treated if they are infected
- Telling sex partners and having them come in to get tested and treated will help stop the spread of this infection

What if I am pregnant or want to get pregnant in the future?
- It is important to get treated for chlamydia *before* you get pregnant
- If you are pregnant and infected with chlamydia, some antibiotics cannot be taken. However, safe, effective treatment with other antibiotics is available to virtually all women
- You and your clinician need to decide on the best treatment for you and your baby
- If untreated, chlamydia before pregnancy can lead to pelvic inflammatory disease, which may cause future infertility

What causes gonorrhea?
- A type of bacteria
- The bacteria can live in the mucus membranes (linings) of the mouth, throat, vagina, cervix, urethra, and rectum
- The infection is spread through oral, genital, or anal contact

What are the symptoms of gonorrhea?
- *Women:* about 50-80% of women do not have any symptoms of infection.
  If there are symptoms they may include unusual discharge from the vagina, burning during urination, or unexplained vaginal bleeding between periods. In later infection they may include pain in lower abdomen, bleeding between periods, or low-grade fever
- *Men:* more likely than women to have symptoms of infection, including watery discharge from the penis, itching or burning around the urethra, or pain when urinating. If untreated, other symptoms may include thick yellow or green discharge from penis, more pain during urination, pain and swelling of the testicles, or low-grade fever (the last two symptoms may mean the man has *epididymitis*, an infection that causes the epididymis (structure in the testicles that stores sperm) to get inflamed)
- If untreated, gonorrhea can lead to serious problems for women such as pelvic inflammatory disease, ectopic pregnancy, or infertility or a more generalized illness for both men and women with a high fever and swollen joints

How will I be tested for gonorrhea?
- A sample is taken using a cervical or penile swab
- A laboratory test is used to look for the bacteria under a microscope
- It is common to test for both gonorrhea and chlamydia

How will I be treated for gonorrhea?
- Treated with antibiotics (e.g., azithromycin, doxycycline, cefixime) taken orally in one dose or for 7-14 days. Frequently, antibiotics will be given as an injection
- Gonorrhea infection of the throat is more difficult to treat than genital infection (similar drugs are used)

What about my sex partner(s)?
- All people with whom you have had sexual contact in the past 60 days need to get tested and treated if they are infected
- Telling sex partners and having them come in to get tested and treated will help stop the spread of this infection

What if I am pregnant or want to get pregnant in the future?
- It is important to get treated for gonorrhea *before* you get pregnant
- If you are pregnant and infected with gonorrhea, some antibiotics cannot be taken. However, safe, effective treatment with other antibiotics is available to virtually all women
- You and your clinician need to decide on the best treatment for you and your baby
- If untreated, gonorrhea can lead to pelvic inflammatory disease, which may cause infertility

STI's Which Tend to Cause Vaginal Discharge

BACTERIAL VAGINOSIS (BV) (bac-TEER-ee-ul va-ji-NO-sis)

NOTE: Bacterial vaginosis is not necessarily a sexually transmitted infection

What causes bacterial vaginosis?
- Most commonly caused by a type of bacteria. Infection occurs when the normal bacteria in the vagina is replaced with an infection-causing bacteria
- It may be transmitted through penile-vaginal intercourse
- It may also arise spontaneously; the causes are not fully understood
- Bacterial vaginosis is the most common cause of vaginal discharge or odor (see symptoms below)
- Bacterial vaginosis is often mistaken for a yeast infection. Therefore, it is important to check with your clinician if you have these symptoms

What are the symptoms of bacterial vaginosis?
- *Women:* 50% of women do not have any symptoms. If there are symptoms, they may include itching, irritation, or white vaginal discharge with a fishy smell
- *Men:* most do not have any symptoms. If there are symptoms, they may include irritation around the urethra and on the head of the penis

How will I be tested for bacterial vaginosis?
- During a pelvic exam, your clinician will check for three of the following signs:
  1.) A white discharge that covers the walls of the vagina
  2.) "Clue cells" in a vaginal smear examined under a microscope
  3.) A high pH of vaginal fluid
  4.) A fishy odor before or after a solution containing 10% potassium hydroxide is added (often a woman notices this right after sex)

How will I be treated for bacterial vaginosis?
- Treated with antibiotics (e.g., metronidazole, clindamycin) taken orally or as a vaginal suppository at bedtime
- ***Do not drink alcohol if you are taking metronidazole or you may become very ill***
- ***Clindamycin cream is oil-based and might weaken latex condoms and diaphragms***
- Return to your clinician if your symptoms do not go away after treatment

What about my sex partner(s)?
- In studies, treatment of male sex partners has not been beneficial in preventing the recurrence of bacterial vaginosis

What if I am pregnant or want to get pregnant in the future?
- Bacterial vaginosis can cause problems in pregnancy (your water may break too early and you may have preterm (early) labor and birth). It may also cause an infection in the uterus after birth
- Because treatment of BV in women at a high risk of pregnancy problems (especially women who have previously delivered a premature baby) who do not have any symptoms might reduce preterm delivery, such women may be screened, and those with BV can be treated. Screening and treatment (with an antibiotic such as metronidazole or clindamycin) should be conducted at the earliest part of the second trimester of pregnancy
- Low-risk pregnant women (e.g., those who previously have not delivered a premature baby) who have symptomatic BV should be treated with antibiotics to relieve the symptoms
- If you are concerned about BV infection during pregnancy, discuss this with your clinician

TRICHOMONIASIS (trik-o-mo-NY-a-sis), or "trich"

What causes trichomoniasis?
- A type of parasite
- It is usually passed through vaginal and anal sexual intercourse
- It can also be passed on dirty towels or washcloths (but this is not common)

What are the symptoms of trichomoniasis?
- ***Women:*** intense itching of vagina and vulva, frothy, fishy-smelling vaginal discharge, or painful intercourse
- ***Men:*** most men do not have any symptoms. If they do have symptoms, they may include painful urination, frequent urination, or white or yellow discharge from the penis

How will I be tested for trichomoniasis?
- A laboratory test is used to look for the parasite under a microscope

How will I be treated for trichomoniasis?
- Treated with antibiotics (e.g. metronidazole) taken orally in a single dose or for 7 days
- Studies on treatments have shown that metronidazole is 90-95% effective in treating trichomoniasis

What about my sex partner(s)?
- All people with whom you have had sexual contact in the past month need to get tested and treated if they are infected
- Telling sex partners and having them go to a clinic to get tested and treated will help stop the spread of this infection

What if I am pregnant or want to get pregnant in the future?
- There is a risk of problems during pregnancy if trichomoniasis is not treated. Your water may break too early and you may have preterm (early) labor and birth
- Tell your clinician if you are pregnant so you can be treated as soon as possible

CANDIDIASIS (YEAST INFECTION) (kan-di-DI-a-sis)

NOTE: Yeast infection is usually not acquired through sexual intercourse

What causes a yeast infection?
- Usually caused by a type of yeast called *Candida albicans*
- The yeast is normally found in the vagina, but sometimes certain conditions cause it to multiply very quickly, causing a yeast infection from overgrowth
- The factors that contribute to recurrent yeast infections are not fully understood. Some possible explanations include: diabetes, having a disease that weakens the immune system, and using steriods
- Yeast infection is common. About 75% of women will have at least one yeast infection in their lives. Probably less than 5% of women will have yeast infections that come back regularly

What are the symptoms of a yeast infection?
- **Women:** intense itching of the vulva and vagina; a white, lumpy discharge from the vagina that may look like cottage cheese; discomfort during intercourse; soreness or burning in the vagina; or burning during urination
- **Men:** may not have any symptoms or may have pain or burning during urination, sores on the penis, or inflammation of the tip of the penis

How will I be tested for a yeast infection?
- If you are not sure you have a yeast infection, it is a good idea to get a clinical exam
- Your clinician will probably look for the yeast under a microscope after taking a swab of your discharge
- About 10-20% of women have yeast without having symptoms so your clinician needs to take your symptoms into consideration when you are diagnosed

How will I be treated for a yeast infection?
- You can buy medicine over the counter at drug stores (e.g., Monistat, Gyne-Lotrimin). These are vaginal creams and suppositories. They cost $12-$20
- Creams are used on the outside of the vagina to stop the itching. Gel applicators or suppositories are put into the vagina at night to kill the yeast
- Prescription drugs are also available from your clinician in the form of creams, suppositories, and pills that you take orally (e.g., clotrimazole, miconazole, terconazole, ketaconazole, fluconazole)
- *NOTE: Creams and suppositories are oil-based and should not be used with condoms because they weaken the latex and may cause condoms to break*
- Some of the oral drugs (especially Ketaconazole) may cause problems if taken with other drugs (Viagra, some heart medicines, and anything that contains nitric oxide). Ask your clinician if you are worried about a potentially dangerous combination

- Maintaining a good level of basic genital and general health may help prevent yeast infections. Use a mild soap and wipe from front to back with toilet papler to avoid bringing bowel bacteria into your vaginal area. Wear cotton underpants. Avoid nylon pantyhose and underpants, and very tight jeans or pants, because they tend to hold moisture in the vaginal area. Avoid bubble baths, bath oils, and hygiene sprays. Avoid douching, which can irritate the vaginal lining making you more vulnerable to infection. Avoid deodorant tampons and pads. Lose weight if you are overweight (extra pounds means the vulva has less exposure to air). Avoid using petroleum jelly lubricants such as Vaseline during sex because they tend to say in the vagina, are hard to wash away and may even promote infection. Infections also seem to occur more frequently during stressful times. Try to maintain a healthy physical and emotional balance in your life and you may experience fewer infections. *[Stewart, Guest, Stewart, Hatcher, 1987]*
- Return to your clinician if your symptoms do not get better after treatment

What about my sex partner(s)?
- Usually your sex partners do not have to be tested or treated. Yeast infection is not usually sexually transmitted. If male sex partners do have symptoms of infection, they may benefit from treatment and should see a clinician

What if I am pregnant or want to get pregnant in the future?
- Many women get yeast infections during pregnancy
- Only medicines such as creams and suppositories should be used to treat yeast infections in pregnant women
- The most effective treatments are butoconazole, clotrimazole, miconazole, and terconazole (all prescription medicines you can get from your clinician)
- Many experts recommend treatment for 7 days during pregnancy

Other STIs

PELVIC INFLAMMATORY DISEASE (PID)

What causes pelvic inflammatory disease (PID)?
- Caused by an infection in the the fallopian tubes and ovaries
- Sexually transmitted infections that do not get treated (such as chlamydia and gonorrhea) are often the cause of PID
- **PID can cause scarring in the fallopian tubes, which may lead to infertility** (not being able to get pregnant)

What are the symptoms of PID?
- Pain or tenderness in the lower abdomen and pelvic area
- Fever and/or chills
- Abnormal vaginal discharge
- Some women may not have any symptoms

How will I get tested for PID?
- You need to be examined immediately by a clinician if you have any of the above symptoms
- If no other cause for the illness can be found and you have pain or tenderness in the lower abdomen or pelvic area, you will most likely be diagnosed with PID

How will I be treated for PID?
- Treated with antibiotics (e.g., clindamycin, metronidazole, oflxacin, cefotetan, doxycycline) taken orally, via intramuscular injection, or, in the hospital, through an IV (a needle put in your vein)
- If PID is severe, you may need to stay in the hospital. The following reasons may require a hospital stay:
  - If a surgical emergency such as appendicitis cannot be excluded as a cause of the symptoms
  - You are pregnant
  - Oral antibiotics are not effective in treating the infection
  - You are unable to take the antibiotics on your own
  - You have a severe illness, nausea or vomiting, or a high fever
  - You have a tuboovarian abscess (an infected, pus-filled area on the fallopian tubes or ovaries)
  - You have a problem with your immune system (you are HIV-positive, taking drugs that affect the immune system, or have another disease)
  - You are a teenager

What about my sex partner(s)?
- Any sex partners with whom you have had contact may be infected with a sexually transmitted infection such as chlamydia or gonorrhea
- It is important to tell your sex partners so that they can be tested and treated if they are infected

What if I am pregnant or want to get pregnant in the future?
- If you are pregnant and have PID, you need to stay in the hospital so you can be given IV antibiotics

What causes HPV?

- A virus called the human papilloma virus (HPV)
- There are approximately 20 types of HPV. Each has been given a number and has a different effect on the body
- Sometimes (but not always) HPV causes genital warts on or around the vagina, penis, or anus or inside the vagina, cervix, or rectum
- HPV is passed by coming into contact with infected skin or mucus membranes
- HPV is one of the most common sexually transmitted infections

What are the symptoms of HPV?

- Most types of HPV do not cause any symptoms
- Visible genital warts are usually caused by types 6 or 11
- Genital warts come in different shapes and sizes. Some are flat, while others are raised or look bumpy like little cauliflowers
- Other types of HPV (types 16, 18, 31, 33, and 35) have been associated with cervical dysplasia (abnormal cell growth on the cervix that can eventually lead to cancer)

How will I be tested for HPV?

- If you have visible warts on the external genitals, your clinician may be able to diagnose you by examining the warts
- An internal exam may be needed to see warts on the inside of the vagina or rectum
- Sometimes a clinician will apply a vinegar solution to the area. If certain areas turn white it could mean you have HPV infection
- It is not necessary for your clinician to identify the type of HPV in diagnosing and treating visible genital warts
- HPV has been linked to cervical dysplasia—a precancerous condition that can develop into cancer if it is not treated right away. Therefore, it is very important that you have regular gynecological exams and Pap tests. The Pap test is not a test specifically for HPV, but if cervical dysplasia is detected on your Pap, it may mean that you are infected with HPV. If you do have dysplasia, there are treatments available to remove the abnormal cells. (NOTE: A Pap test is different from a pelvic exam, although they may be done at the same time. During a Pap test, your clinician takes a swab of the cells on the cervix, which are then tested in a lab.) It is a screening test for cervical cancer

How will I be treated for HPV?

- **There is no cure for HPV.** Visible warts can be treated but no evidence indicates that currently available treatments eliminate HIV. The removal of warts may or may not decrease your ability to transmit the infection to partners
- Warts can be removed by cryotherapy (freezing), laser therapy (burning), or applying a chemical solution to kill the warts
- In some treatments you will put on the medicine (a cream) yourself at bedtime
- Treatment of warts inside the rectum should be referred to an expert
- If left untreated, visible warts may go away on their own, remain unchanged, or increase in size and number
- Treatment usually causes wart-free periods in most people, but warts can come back again
- No evidence indicates that treatment of visible warts affects the development of cervical cancer
- **You can transmit the infection to others even after the warts are removed because the virus remains in your body**

What about my sex partner(s)?
- Sex partners who have visible warts need to be treated
- Examination of sex partner without symptoms is not necessary because the role of reinfection is probably minimal and, because there is no cure for HPV, treatment to reduce transmission is not realistic. However, because it may be difficult to recognize warts if they are present, an exam with a clinician may help sex partners identify warts or other STIs
- Because treatment of genital warts probably does not eliminate the HPV infection, it is important to know that you may be able to spread HPV even after warts are removed. The use of condoms may reduce, but does not eliminate, the risk of transmission to uninfected partners
- Female sex partners who have genital warts need to have regular Pap tests to screen for cervical cancer (as do all sexually active women)

What if I am pregnant or want to get pregnant in the future?
- Some treatments (e.g., imiquimod, podophyllin, and podofilox) should not be used during pregnancy
- Genital warts can increase during pregnancy, so most experts recommend that they be treated
- Passed from mother to child, HPV types 6 and 11 rarely can infect children in the throat. The specifics of transmission are not yet fully understood
- If HPV causes cervical dysplasia that develops into cancer, a woman can have problems during pregnancy and birth

STI's Which Are Preventable With Vaccines

HEPATITIS A and B (hep-a-TI-tis)

What causes hepatitis?

- A type of virus
- There are two types of hepatitis that we will discuss here: A and B. Hepatitis A is most commonly passed through oral contact with infected fecal matter (stool) either by person-to-person transmission between household contacts or sex partners or by contaminated food or water. Hepatitis B is usually passed through sexual activity (through blood, semen, saliva, vaginal fluids, urine, and fecal matter). Hepatitis B may also be passed from a pregnant mother to her infant (risk is 10-85% and depends on the status of the mother's immune system)
- Hepatitis A and B attack the liver and the illness can be very serious

What are the symptoms of hepatitis?

- Fatigue (feeling tired)
- Diarrhea
- Nausea and vomiting
- Abdominal pain
- Jaundice (yellowish skin or eyes)
- Dark yellow or orange urine

How will I be tested for hepatitis?

- A blood test is used to identify the virus

How will I be treated for hepatitis?

- There is no specific medical treatment for hepatitis A or B—the illness has to run its course
- Usually, infected people need to rest and drink lots of fluids for a couple of weeks
- Sometimes the infection is serious and you may need to stay in the hospital
- Liver damage or death may result in severe cases (about 6,000 people die each year from hepatitis)
- Once you recover you cannot get infected again with hepatitis A. Infection with Hepatitis B may result in recovery or it may become a chronic disease
- **The best way to prevent hepatitis is to get vaccinated against it (a series of 3 shots over 6 months for hepatitis B and 2 vaccines 6 months apart for hepatitis A)—ask your clinician today about these simple and effective vaccines**

What about my sex partner(s)?

- Sex partners or other people recently exposed to Hepatitis A (e.g., through household contact) and who have not been vaccinated before the exposure should receive a vaccine, but not if it has been more than 14 days after exposure
- Sex partners should be immunized with hepatitis B immune globulin (HBIG) and begin the vaccine series within 14 days after the most recent sexual contact

What if I am pregnant or want to get pregnant in the future?

- Pregnant women should be tested for hepatitis infection
- Pregnant women can still be vaccinated against hepatitis

STI's Which are Caused by Parasites

PUBIC LICE, or "crabs"

What causes pubic lice?
- A type of parasite
- It is passed through sexual contact or from using sheets, toilet seats, underwear or other clothes, or towels that have lice on them (lice can live up to one day and lay eggs without being on a human)
- Female lice lay eggs which hatch in 7-9 days and begin laying their own eggs in about 2 weeks

What are the symptoms of pubic lice?
- Itching in the pubic area, especially in the hair
- You may be able to see the lice or eggs on your pubic hair close to the skin

How will I be tested for pubic lice?
- A clinician can examine you to see if lice or eggs are found

How will I be treated for pubic lice?
- Over-the-counter medicines come in the form of shampoo or lotion (e.g., Kwell, Nix, RID)
- Prescription medicines are also available from your clinician and come in the form of shampoo (e.g., permethrin, lindane)
- You will need to wash all of your bedding and clothing (either machine-wash and dry them using the heat cycle or have them dry cleaned)
- It is not necessary to fumigate living areas

What about my sex partner(s)?
- All people with whom you have had sexual contact in the past month need to be treated if they are infected
- Telling sex partners and having them get treated will help stop the spread of this infection

What if I am pregnant or want to get pregnant in the near future?
- The prescription medicine, Lindane, should not be used by pregnant or breastfeeding women
- Talk to your clinician about the best treatment for you

NOTE: Scabies is not necessarily a sexually transmitted infection.

What causes scabies?

- A type of parasite
- Parasites tunnel underneath the skin to lay their eggs and the immature parasites make their way back to the surface, causing skin irritation
- Scabies is very contagious. It is passed easily between people in close contact (sexually and nonsexually)
- Scabies can infect many body areas, including the genitals, buttocks, feet, wrists, hands, abdomen, armpits, or scalp

What are the symptoms of scabies?

- Intense itching with or without a red rash

How will I be tested for scabies?

- A clinician can examine you to see if the parasites are found

How will I be treated for scabies?

- Usually treated with prescription medicines available from your provider that come in the form of lotion (e.g., permethrin, lindane)
- You will need to wash all of your bedding and clothing (either machine-wash and dry them using the heat cycle or have them dry cleaned)
- It is not necessary to fumigate living areas

What about my sex partner(s)?

- All people with whom you have had close contact (sexual and non-sexual close contact, including household contact) in the past month need to be treated if they are infected
- Telling sex partners and having them get treated will help stop the spread of this infection

What if I am pregnant or want to get pregnant in the near future?

- The prescription medicine, Lindane, should not be used by pregnant or breastfeeding women
- Talk to your clinician about the best treatment for you

"Women Hold Up Half the Sky"

This Chinese and African proverb crosses all cultural boundaries. Actually it is sometimes put this way: Women hold up *more* than half the sky. It represents one of the most important messages about family planning: If human beings are to make true progress in the most important health problems facing the world—maternal mortality, deaths from unsafe abortion, teenage pregnancy, HIV infection, infertility, family planning and slowing population growth—the status of women MUST improve.

In many cultures and societies throughout history, other people and institutions have controlled the reproductive lives of women. For today's contraceptive technologies to meet their full potential, women must be able to hold their reproductive destinies.

A fundamental part of improving the status of women is male involvement in family planning. It is a myth that contraception is only a woman's responsibility. After all, it takes both a man and a woman to create life; it also takes both a man and a woman to plan families and prevent unintended pregnancies.

Although there are currently many contraceptive methods for women, two of the best methods are for men: vasectomy and condoms. Vasectomy is safer, cheaper, and more effective than tubal ligation (female sterilization). Condoms are cheap, readily available, and help protect against unintended pregnancy and sexually transmitted infections.

When Bob Hatcher was on Ted Kopel's NIGHTLINE he was asked for a final comment. He said, "For all too long, the reproductive destinies of women have been controlled by popes, presidents and politicians, usually men. This must stop."

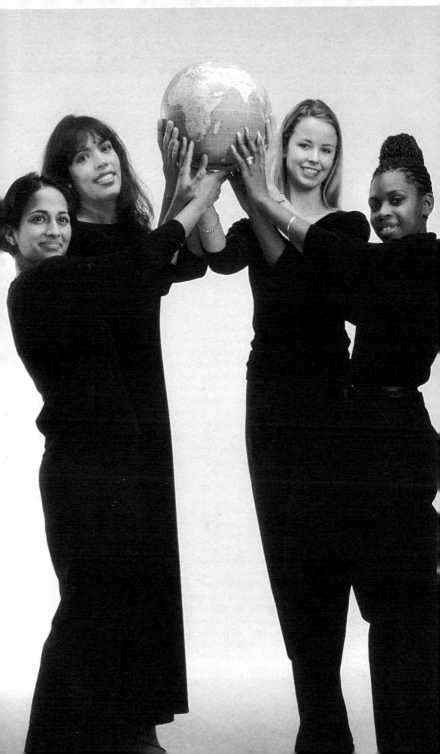

"Human needs will not be met without more concerned action on human numbers."

—PROFESSOR JOHN GUILLEBAUD

2000	Estimated world population: 6,165,485,000
1999	World population hits **6 billion** (this billion took 12 years)
1997	FDA approves Emergency Contraceptive Pills
1994	Plastic (polyurethane) condom for men (Avanti)
1993	FDA approves polyurethane (plastic) female condom (Reality)
1993	Researchers Creinin and Darney describe medical abortion using methotrexate
1992	FDA approves Depo-Provera (DMPA) injections
1990	FDA approves Norplant implants
1988	Copper T 380-A IUD marketing begins, 5 years after FDA approval
1987	World population reaches **5 billion** (this billion took 12 years)
1983	FDA approves Copper T 380-A and the Today sponge
1982	Researcher Baulieu describes medical abortion using mifepristone
1981	First recognized case of HIV/AIDS
1981	Garret Hardin sarcastically writes "nobody ever dies of overpopulation" after 500,000 die from flooding of an overcrowded East Bengal River delta
1975	World population reaches **4 billion** (this billion took 15 years)
1974	Al Yuzpe describes emergency contraception using Ovral pills
1973	FDA approved progestin-only pills (minipills)
1973	U.S. Supreme Court abortion decision (Roe v Wade)
1965	U.S. Supreme Court decision overturns anti-birth control laws in most states (Griswold v. CT)
1965	U.S. Agency for International Development initiates Population Program
1960	Food and Drug Administration approves combined oral contraceptives
1960	World population reaches **3 billion** (this billion took 30 years)
1942	American Birth Control League renamed Planned Parenthood
1937	American Medical Association ends longstanding opposition to contraception
1936	German gynecologist Friedrich Wilde describes first cervical cap (fitted from a wax impression)
1930-31	Knaus (Austria) and Ogino (Japan) develop rhythm method
1930	World population now **2 billion** (this billion took 100 years)
1930	Pope Pius XI strongly attacks both contraception & abortion
1927	Novak (Hopkins) describes suction as a way of performing an abortion
1916	Margaret Sanger opens first Amercian birth control clinic in Brooklyn, NY
1914	Margaret Sanger coins word "birth control"
1912	Sadie Sachs dies from abortion and drives Margaret Sanger to advocate safe birth control
1909	German surgeon Richard Richter reports success with silkworm-gut shaped into a ring as an IUD
1904	Basal body temperature fluctuations described
1893	First vasectomy
1882	First contraceptive clinic established in Amsterdam
1880	First tubal ligation sterilization
1873	Comstock Act: classifies all images of contraception as obscene
1839	Charles Goodyear discovers vulcanization technology; quickly leads to rubber condoms
1830	World population reaches **1 billion** (this billion took 6 million years)
1798	Thomas Robert Malthus proposes dismal theory that population growth eventually will exceed the ability of the earth to provide food, resulting in starvation
Late 1770s	Casanova popularizes condoms for infection control and contraception
1 AD	World population reaches **250 million**. To control births, people use abstinence (especially after birth), withdrawal, breastfeeding, stones in camels, lemons to block and kill sperm, and abortion using molokeeia (same stem used today)

Side annotations:
- **1999 - 6 billion people (10/12/99)**
- **1987 - 5 billion people**
- **1975 - 4 billion people**
- **1960 - 3 billion people**
- **1930 - 2 billion people**
- **1800 - 1 billion people**
- **1 AD - 250 million people**

Special thanks to Andrea Tone at Georgia Tech

American College of Obstetrics and Gynecologists (ACOG). Emergency oral contraception. ACOG Practice Patterns 1996 (Dec. no. 3).

Anderson K. Personal communication to Hatcher RA. National Medical Committee of the Planned Parenthood Federation of America, 1997 Aug 12.

Berel V, Hermon C, Kay C, Hannaford P, Darby S, Reeves G. Mortality associated with oral contraceptive use: 25 year follow-up of cohort of 46,000 women from Royal College of General Practitioners' oral contraceptive study; Br Med J 1999: 918:96-100.

Brache V, Alvarez-Sanchez F, Faundes A, Tejada AS, Cochon L. Ovarian endocrine function through five years of continuous treatment with Norplant subdermal contraceptive implants. Contraception 1990;41:169.

Centers for Disease Control and Prevention. 1998 Guidelines for treatment of sexually transmitted diseases. MMWR 1998;47(No. RR-1).

Chandra. National Center for Health Statistics 1998.

Creinin MD. personal communication to Hatcher RA, Feb. 26, 1999.

Creinin MD, Burke AE. Methotrexate and misoprostol for early abortion: a multicenter trial. Acceptability. Contraception 1996;54:19-22.

Creinin MD, Vittinghoff E, Schaff E, Klaisle C, Darney PD, Dean C. Medical abortion with oral methotrexate and vaginal misoprostol. Obstet Gynecol 1997;90:611-5.

Cromer BA, Blair JM, Mahan JD, Zibners L, Naumovski Z. A prospective comparison of bone density in adolescent girls receiving depo-medroxyprogesteroneacetate (Depo-Provera), levonorgestrel (Norplant), or oral contraceptives. J Pediatr 1996;129:671-6.

Croxatto HB, Diaz S, Pavez M, et al. Plasma progesterone levels during long-term treatment with levonorgestrel silastic implants. Acta Endocrinol 1982;101:307-11.

Farley TM, Rosenberg MS, Rowe PJ, Chen SH, Meirck O. Intrauterine devices and pelvic inflammatory disease: an international perspective. Lancet 1992; 339: 785-88.

Feldblum PJ, Morrison CS, Roddy RE, Cates W Jr. The effectiveness of barrier methods of contraception in preventing the spread of HIV. AIDS 1995;9 (suppl A):585-93.

Food and Drug Administration, 1997.

Fraser SI, Affandi B, Croxatto HB, et al. Norplant consensus statement and background paper. Turku, Finland: Leiras Oy International, 1997.

Goldstein M, Girardi S. Vasectomy and vasectomy reversal. Curr Thera Endocrinol Metab 1997;6:371-80.

Gray RH, Campbell OM, Zacur H, Labbok MH, MacRae SL. Postpartum return of ovarian activity in non-breastfeeding women monitored by urinary assays. J Clin Endocrinol Metab 1987;64:645-50.

Grimes DA. Modern IUDs: an update. The Contraception Report; November, 1998

Haffner DW, Schwartz P. What I've Learned about Sex. A Perigee Book: New York: The Berkeley Publishing Group, 1998.

Hakim-Elahi E, Tovell HMM, Burnhill MS. Complications of first-trimester abortion: a report of 170,000 cases. Obstet Gynecol 1990;76:129.

Henshaw SK. Unintended pregnancy in the United States. Fam Plann Perspect 1998;30:24-9, 46.

Hogue CJR, Cates W Jr, Tietze C. The effects of induced abortion on subsequent reproduction. The Johns Hopkins University School of Hygiene and Public Health. Epidemiol Rev 1982;4:66 International Planned Parenthood Federation Handbook 1997.

Kaunitz AM. personal communication; December 28, 1998 and February 24, 1999.

Kennedy KI, Trussell J. Postpartum contraception and lactation. IN Hatcher RA, Trussell J, Stewart F et al: Contraceptive Technology, 17th ed.; New York: Ardent Media Inc; 1998: 592-4. [The same data are presented in the Family Health International Module for the teaching of Lactational Amenorrhea]

Kjos SL, Peters RK, Xiang A, Duncan T, Schaefer U, Buchanan TA. Contraception and the risk of type 2 diabetes mellitus in Latina women with prior gestational diabetes mellitus. JAMA 1998; 280: 533-38.

Klavon SL, Grubb G. Insertion site complications during the first year of Norplant use. Contraception 1990;41:27.

Narod ST. The Hereditary Ovarian Cancer Clinical Study Group. Oral contraceptives and the risk of hereditary ovarian cancer. N Engl J Med 1998;339;424-8.

Peipert JF, Gutman J. Oral contraceptive risk assessment: a survey of 247 educated women. Obstet Gynecol 1993;82:112-7.

Peterson HB. Lecture on tubal sterilization. Emory University 1998 July 29.

Peterson HB, Pollack AE, Warshaw JS. Tubal sterilization. In: Rock JA, Thompson JD, eds. TeLinde's Operative Gynecology. 8th ed. Philadelphia: Lippincott-Raven, 1997:541-5.

Pfizer's Letter to the Physician. New York: Pfizer Labs, 1998.

Raudaskoski TH, Lahti EI, Kauppila AJ, Apaja-Sarkkinen MA, Laatikainen TJ. Transdermal estrogen with a levonorgestrel-releasing intrauterine device for climacteric complaints: clinical and endometrial responses. Am J Obstet Gynecol 1995;172:114-9.

The Alan Guttmacher Institute. Sex and America's Teenagers. New York and Washington: 1994.

Silvestre L, Dubois C, Renault M, Rezvani Y, Baulieu E, Ulmann A. Voluntary interruption of pregnancy with mifepristone (RU-486) and a prostaglandin analogue. N Engl J Med 1990; 322:645-8.

Smith TW. Personal communication to James Trussell. December 13, 1993.

Speroff L. The perimenospaausal transition: maximizing preventive health care. In: Mooney B, Daughtery J, eds. Midlife Women's Health Sourcebook. Atlanta: American Health Consultants, 1995.

Task Force on Postovulatory Methods of Fertility Regulation. Randomized controlled trial of levonorgestrel versus the Yuzpe regimen of combined oral contraceptives for emergency contraception. Lancet 1998;352:420-33.

The Hereditary Ovarian Cancer Clinical Study Group. Oral contraceptives and the risk of hereditary ovarian cancer. N Engl J Med 1998;339;424-8.

Trussell J, Leveque JA, Koenig JD, et al. The economic value of contraception: a comparison of 15 methods. Am J Public Health 1995;85:494-503.

Trussell J, Stewart F, Guest F, Hatcher RA. Emergency contraceptive pills: a simple proposal to reduce unintended pregnancies. Fam Plann Perspect 1992;24:269-73.

Viagra (sildenafil citrate) tablets. New York: Pfizer Labs, 1998.

White MK, Ory HW, Rooks JB, Rochat RW. Intrauterine device termination rates and menstrual cycle day of insertion. Obstet Gynecol 1980; 55:220-4.

World Health Organization. WHO Taskforce Postovulatory Methods of Fertility Regulation. Lancet Aug 8, 1998.

SPANISH/ESPAÑOL

- Abstinencia
- Amamantando a Su Bebe
- Capuchon Cervical
- Retraer el pene antes de ejecular
- Condones para hombres
- Condones para Mujeres
- El Diafragma
- Contraceptivo de Emergencia
- Las Pastillas Contraceptivo
- Las Pastillas de Progesterona solamente
- El Dispositivo de Cobre "T 380 A"
- Los Metodos Naturales
  El Conocimiento de las Fertilidad
- Espermicidas
- Espuma Contraceptivo
- Tela Contraceptivo
- Gelatina Contraceptivo or Jaleas
- Inyecciones Combinadas
- Inyecciones de Depo-Provera
- Implantes de NORPLANT
- Dispositivos Intrauterinos
- El Dispositivo con "Levo Norgestrel"
- El Dispositivo con "Progestasert"
- Ligadura o Esterilizacion de las Trompas
- Vasectomia

ENGLISH/(INGLES)

- Abstinence
- Breastfeeding
- Cervical Cap
- Coitus Interruptus (Withdrawal)
- Condoms for Men
- Condoms for Women
- Diaphragm
- Emergency Contraception
- Combined Oral Contraceptives
- Progestin-Only Pills
- Copper T 380-A
- Fertility Awareness Methods

- Spermicides
- Foam
- VCF
- Jellies
- Combined Injectables
- Depo-Provera
- Norplant Implant
- IUDs
- Levonorgestrel IUD
- Progestasert IUD
- Tubal Sterilization
- Vasectomy

P

Packard Foundation, ii, xi
PAP test, 172
Pelvic inflammatory disease (PID), 34, 36, 79, 80, 88, 174
Phone numbers, xi
    depression, xi
    emergency contraception, xi, 68
    HIV, xi, 161
    Natural family planning, 47
    Norplant removal, 141
    STIs, xi, 161
Placebo pills, 91, 97
PLAN B, 68-75, 124
Population growth, A-1
Postcoital contraception
    see emergency contraception
Pregnancy
    and adolescents, 18
    and STIs, 1608
    planning, 21-22
    testing, 23
    termination, 25-31
Pregnancy test, 23
Premature ejaculation
    see early ejaculation
Premenstrual Syndrome, 6, 97
Preorgasmia, 12
Preven, 68-74, 76, 124
Progesterone, 5-6
    Progestasert IUD, 85
Progestin, 68-69, 75, 91-97, 118, 126, 135, 136
Progestin-only methods
    see also *Depo-Provera*, Levonorgestrel IUD, *Progestasert* IUD, *Norplant*, and Progestin-only pills
Progestin-only pills
    advantages, 91
    and breastfeeding, 24, 43, 92
    and fertility, 94
    who can use, 93
    risks, 92
    cost, 91
    disadvantages, 92
    effectiveness, 35, 91
    starting method, 93
    what happens if, 94
    Spanish, A-3

R

Rape, ix, xi, 14, 38
RU-486, 29, 30, 77

S

Scabies, 179
Seizures, 93, 101
Sexual assault, ix, xi, 38
Sexual behavior, 8, 10-17
Sexual dysfunction, 11-17
Sexual history, 10
Sexually transmissible infections (STIs), 158-179
    see specific infection
    see p.158 for table of contents of STI section
    adolescents, 18, 160
    cervical cap, 56, 159
    combined oral contraceptive, 97, 159
    diaphragm, 59, 159
    female condom, 53, 159
    IUDs, 78, 159
    male condom, 48, 159
    pregnancy, 21, 160
    prevention method, 160
    spermicides, 62, 159
    withdrawal, 66, 159
Sickle cell disease, 22
Smoking and contraception, 100, 104, 106
Spanish, A-3
Sperm, 3, 48, 53, 56, 59, 62, 64, 66, 78, 91, 97, 126, 136, 151
Spermicides, 62-65
    advantages, 62-63
    and fertility, 64
    and other contraceptives, 48, 63, 159
    and STIs, 62, 63, 159
    who can use, 63
    risks, 36, 48, 63
    cost, 62
    disadvantages, 36, 62-63
    effectiveness, 35, 62
    foam, 62
    starting method, 63
    noncontraceptive benefits, 36, 62
    what happens if, 64
    Spanish, A-3
Sponge, 64-65
STI
    see sexually transmissible infections

**If you have any questions,
ask us at...
www.managingcontraception.com**

Your <u>Personal Guide to Managing Contraception</u> has a sister and a grandfather!

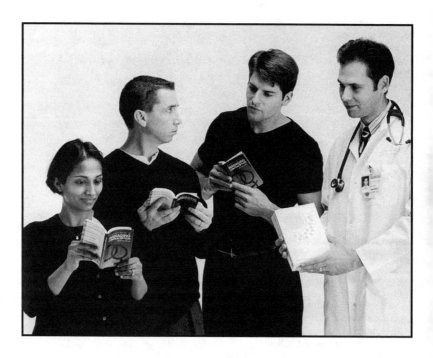

The very, very small sister-book for clinicians, *A Pocket Guide to Managing Contraception*, has exactly the same chapters and content as *A Personal Guide to Managing Contraception*. Both of these small books have a backup reference book, 17 editions since 1969, called *Contraceptive Technology*.

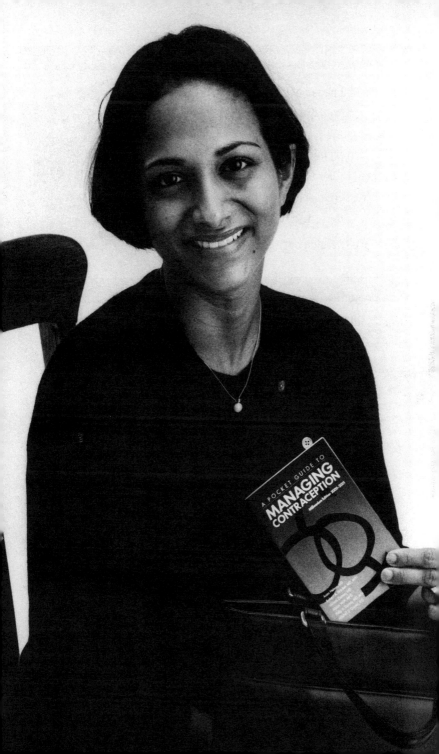

A Pocket Guide to Managing Contraception

Includes 200 pages of information including:

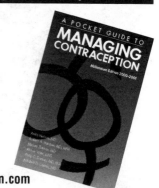

- STI's (CDC Guidelines)
- Depo-Provera (what procedure to follow if late getting injection)
- 8 pages in color of all oral contraceptives
- Menstrual cycle physiology
- and MUCH MORE!

Larger print version available through amazon.com

Contraceptive Technology

Over 1 million copies sold since original printing! A must for every clinic!

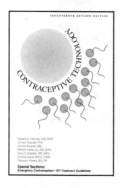

The 17th Edition of *Contraceptive Technology* has drawn on experts throughout the country to author chapters of this <u>NEW</u> book. So it is the BEST EVER!! It includes the 1998 STI guidelines from the CDC. We know you will enjoy this practical reference book.

Actual Size: 6" x 9"
880 pages

The Quest for Excellence

For high school students 13 to 18

The Quest for Excellence is a must for teaching and learning reproductive health. Deals with "How to Say No" and building self-esteem around a healthy sexual identity. For teenagers and parents of teenagers.

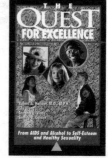

Size: 3.5" x 5.5"
182 pages

Sexual Etiquette 101 & More

For college students & all young adults (18-22)

Includes current information on the following:

- Filled with actual case histories and many illustrations.

- Making a Personal Life Plan, Decision-Making Skills, Developing Self-Esteem, Learning to Communicate

- Your Body, The Menstrual Cycle, Expressing Your Sexuality, Masturbation, Sexual Concerns

- Sexually Transmitted Diseases: What are these and how to protect yourself against them.

- Contraception and Emergency Contraception

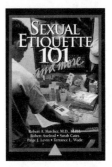

Size: 4.25" x 6.25"
160 pages

Emergency Contraception

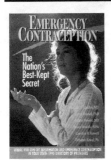

The Nation's Best Kept Secret

Simple, safe, legal and effective emergency contraceptive options are now available. They are described in this 250 page book, written by a team that includes some of the nation's leading contraceptive experts.

Actual Size:
4.25" x 6.25"
250 pages

Something Nice to Do 365 Days a Year

A Convenient Desk Calendar by Robert A. Hatcher, M.D.

This book is more than a desk calendar for the year 2000. It is a book of suggestions of nice things to do...for others, or for yourself. Consider writing down each day something nice you have done for another person or for yourself. Includes wonderful photography for each month of the year!

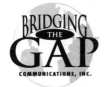

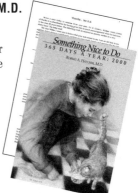

Actual Size:
6" x 9"

Order Form

	Quantity	Total
Personal Guide to Managing Contraception for Women and Men		
1-99 14.95 ea	_____	_____
100-199 11.95 ea	_____	_____
200-299 10.95 ea	_____	_____
Managing Contraception		
1-99 10.00 ea	_____	_____
100-199 9.00 ea	_____	_____
200-299 8.00 ea	_____	_____
Contraceptive Technology - 17th Edition		
1-24 39.95 ea	_____	_____
25-50 35.00 ea	_____	_____
51-100 30.00 ea	_____	_____
Sexual Etiquette 101 & More		
1-24 4.95 ea	_____	_____
25-499 2.00 ea	_____	_____
500-999 1.50 ea	_____	_____
1000 up 1.00 ea	_____	_____
Quest for Excellence		
1-24 4.95 ea	_____	_____
25-499 2.00 ea	_____	_____
500-999 1.50 ea	_____	_____
1000 up 1.00 ea	_____	_____
Emergency Contraception (The Nation's Best Kept Secret)		
1-99 10.00 ea	_____	_____
Something Nice Calender		
1-9 10.00 ea	_____	_____
10-499 8.00 ea	_____	_____
Sub total		_____
Georgia locations add 7% sales tax		_____
Add $1.00 + 15% Shipping & Handling		_____
Total Enclosed		_____

We accept check or credit cards: VISA, MasterCard, Discover, & American Express

Credit Card No. _____ Expiration Date: _____

Signature: _____ (Required)

SHIP TO: Name: _____

Organization: _____

Address: _____

_____ Zip _____

Phone No. _____ Fax No. _____

Mail or Fax this ORDER FORM with your payment to:
Bridging the Gap Communications • P.O. Box 33218 • Decatur, GA 30033
Make checks payable to Bridging the Gap Communications
Phone: (404) 373-0530 • Fax: (404) 373-0480 • www.managingcontraception.com

THANK YOU! (CALL FOR SPECIAL PRICES ON LARGER QUANTITIES & INTERNATIONAL SHIPPING)

JS/RAH/AP 11/99

Did you know that there is a place on the Internet where you can go to ask questions and get answers about contraception? Check out www.managingcontraception.com to ask questions and get answers from medical experts, learn what's new in the world of contraception, order other books about sexual and reproductive health, and print out pages from *A Pocket Guide to Managing Contraception* (a book for health care providers). Here is an example of a recent question and its answer:

Q *"We are considering the IUD as a means of contraception. We are both in late 20s and Jana has not had any children yet. In the future she wants to have children. Is there any significant incidence of decreased fertility in women who have used the IUD? In some materials we have read that some doctors will not prescribe the IUD to women who have not yet had children. What is the reason for this? Are there any other negative side effects of the IUD? Have the negative side effects of the IUDs from the past (like the 70s) been eliminated by the newer generations of IUDs? "*

A The negative side effects of IUDs during the 70s centered upon the Dalkon Shield and its complications. The tail attached to this IUD was entirely different than the tail(s) attached to any other IUDs. Dalkon Shields had a polyfilimented tail consisting of an outer sheath surrounding many very small filaments. The effect of this polyfilimented tail was to draw bacteria from the vagina up into the uterine cavity. It has been called a wicking effect. The active transport system increased by a factor of over 8 a woman's risk for pelvic infections (endometritis, salpingitis or even peritonitis). These tails of other IUDs do not have an active transport system pulling bacteria up into the uterus. The tails of all other IUDs are monofilament tails.

At a recent conference sponsored by The Association of Reproductive Health Professionals, I asked individuals how they would characterize their advice to nulliparous women regarding IUD use. Here is what they said:

I am very comfortable about putting in an IUD for a woman who is not at risk for infections. There is probably a reason why you are wanting to consider an IUD. Perhaps problems with pills. Perhaps an unintended pregnancy leading to an abortion. A number of well-performed studies have concluded that IUDs have not increased tubal occlusion or infertility. The main reason doctors are reluctant regarding IUDs has been the legal climate and awareness that insertions are a bit more difficult and likely to cause more pain. In this setting, I would use a local anesthesia at the time of insertion. (Approximately one out of 10 to one out of 20 IUDs I insert are for nulligravid.)

—Andrew Kaunitz, MD
Professor of Gynecology and Obstetrics
University of Florida (Jacksonville)

For the nulligranda requesting IUD (after understanding all her other options), I spend more time in counseling about future fertility risks associated with exposure to infections. I don't like it for young women with history of serial monogamy, but have placed IUDs in nulligranda women in a stable long-term relationship. I'm not concerned that the IUD itself causes infertility, but that infection risks in an IUD user are the real problem. Therefore, I will place it if the patient and I determine together that she is an appropriate candidate.

—Melisa Holmes, MD
Associate Professor of Obstetrics and Gynecology
Medical University of South Carolina

(MH has inserted 6-7 IUDs for nulliparous women. All have been medical students or residents.)

There is more to this answer on our website:

www.managingcontraception.com